Spiritually Competent Practice in Health Care

Spiritually Competent Practice in Health Care

Edited By

John Wattis
School of Human and Health Sciences
University of Huddersfield
Huddersfield, UK

Stephen Curran
School of Human and Health Sciences
University of Huddersfield
Huddersfield, UK

Melanie Rogers
School of Human and Health Sciences
University of Huddersfield
Huddersfield, UK

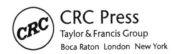

CRC Press
Taylor & Francis Group
Boca Raton London New York

CRC Press is an imprint of the
Taylor & Francis Group, an **informa** business

CRC Press
Taylor & Francis Group
6000 Broken Sound Parkway NW, Suite 300
Boca Raton, FL 33487-2742

© 2017 by Taylor & Francis Group, LLC
CRC Press is an imprint of Taylor & Francis Group, an Informa business

No claim to original U.S. Government works

Printed on acid-free paper

International Standard Book Number-13: 978-1-4987-7842-8 (Paperback)

Library of Congress Cataloging-in-Publication Data

Names: Wattis, John, 1949- editor. | Curran, Stephen, editor. | Rogers, Melanie, editor.
Title: Spiritually competent practice in health care / [edited by] John Wattis, Stephen Curran, Melanie Rogers.
Description: Boca Raton : CRC Press, [2017] | Includes bibliographical references.
Identifiers: LCCN 2016051833 (print) | LCCN 2016052607 (ebook) | ISBN 9781138739116
(hardback : alk. paper) | ISBN 9781498778428 (pbk. : alk. paper) | ISBN 9781315188638 (Master eBook)
Subjects: | MESH: Spirituality | Delivery of Health Care | Holistic Health
Classification: LCC R733 (print) | LCC R733 (ebook) | NLM W 62 | DDC 615.5—dc23
LC record available at https://lccn.loc.gov/2016051833

Visit the Taylor & Francis Web site at
http://www.taylorandfrancis.com

and the CRC Press Web site at
http://www.crcpress.com

Contents

Foreword

The editors have done a fine job of putting together a book that will be of tremendous use to all health care professionals from physicians to nurses to social workers, rehabilitation therapists, and chaplains. The pathway taken here is a sensible and reasonable one, emphasizing a patient-centered approach that underscores the importance of spiritually competent care. They do an excellent job of describing how to integrate spirituality into patient care for all of the different health care professionals. They also emphasize the importance of an evidence-based approach that is guided by research.

Integrating spirituality into patient care is indeed a team effort. No one health care professional has the training or skills or opportunity to do all that is required in order to comprehensively identify and address patients' spiritual needs related to health. Given the many tasks that are now demanded of health care professionals with less and less time to do so, no single health care professional can do all that is required. Each health care professional has a specific job that they are uniquely qualified for in this effort to provide whole-person health care that includes the spiritual component.

Working together with the Adventist Health System, the largest Protestant health care system in the United States and possibly the world, we have developed a practical approach for assessing and addressing patients' spiritual needs in the US health care setting (particularly the outpatient care setting, where chaplains are often not immediately available). We call this the Spiritual Care Team (SCT) approach, which has now been adopted by and assessed in 520 physicians and mid-level providers in outpatient practices across the eastern and midwestern United States. The program has included a research component, where all participants are assessed at baseline, 1 month, and 12 months into the program. The intention is to demonstrate that such a program can impact clinician behavior in a way that is acceptable and satisfying to patients (the results are currently submitted for publication). The Adventist Health System plans to continue this effort into the future in order to carry out its faith-based mission. Nevertheless, there is nothing unique to a faith-based system in this approach, and we believe that this way of assessing and addressing patients' spiritual needs will soon spread to secular health care systems as the benefits to physician well-being, patient satisfaction, and overall health care costs become evident.

In the SCT approach, the physician performs the screening spiritual history (SSH). The SSH consists of three short questions: (1) 'Do you have a faith-based support system to help you in times of need?'; 'Do you have any religious beliefs that might influence your medical decisions?'; and 'Do you have any other spiritual concerns that you would like someone to address?' Patient responses are then documented in the electronic medical record. The training program makes clear to everyone that the physician cannot defer this task of identifying spiritual needs through the SSH to nurses or other team members (which is the temptation here in the United States, where only 10% of clinicians regularly take a spiritual history). We feel that it is essential for the physician to ask these questions because the answers to them relate to medical decisions, and they also send a message to the patient that these issues are important and that they can be discussed if necessary within the clinician.

If spiritual needs are identified by the physician, he or she does not usually have the time or the training to address them, so a spiritual care coordinator (SCC) (usually a nurse or practice manager trained specifically for this purpose) addresses minor spiritual needs that are present, but more than likely will refer all but the most minor issues to a professional chaplain. The chaplain then contacts the patient, conducts a thorough spiritual assessment, comes up with a treatment plan, and communicates their findings and suggestions back to the health care team. This information is then discussed during an SCT meeting that usually occurs about once per month. In this way, information learned by the chaplain that relates to the patient's health care makes it back to the clinicians who can then provide care that is sensitive to the patient's spiritual and cultural background.

A similar approach is being pursued among hospitalized patients, where the physician again is in charge of doing the initial screening and then nurses on the unit contact the chaplain for any spiritual needs that are identified. The chaplain will round with other health care professionals as they visit the patient during the day, offering suggestions as appropriate based on their comprehensive spiritual assessment of the patient that is also documented in the medical record. Occupational and physical therapists can utilize this information as well, or conduct their own brief spiritual history in order to develop a rehabilitation program that is sensitive to the patient's spiritual needs. The social worker also serves an important role in this setting as he or she works with the chaplain to help provide follow-up after the patient is discharged from the hospital.

In order to identify the benefits of this approach and other approaches described in this book, as the authors indicate, it is essential that such interventions are guided by systematic research that assesses both patient and clinician responses to such programs. While qualitative evidence from single or multiple case reports is important and useful for developing and fine-tuning any attempts to assess and address patients' spiritual needs, it is not sufficient. Those who run the health care system do so using numbers. Clinicians learn about treatments and interventions from quantitative studies published in medical and nursing journals. Thus, quantitative systematic research is necessary in the education of both health care professionals and hospital administrators, who are used to making decisions based on numbers. If benefits to health care professionals and patients can be demonstrated by quantitative research that is generalizable to all patients, then it is likely that such programs will receive the support necessary that will enable them to endure over the long term.

Thus, I am excited to see that efforts are being made in the European setting to identify, support, and address patients' spiritual needs as they relate to health care, and to do so in a competent manner that is patient centered, practical, and sensible. This book provides superb guidelines that will be enormously helpful to every health care professional.

Harold G Koenig, MD
Professor of Psychiatry & Behavioral Sciences
Associate Professor of Medicine
Director, Center for Spirituality, Theology and Health
Duke University Medical Center, Durham, North Carolina
Adjunct Professor, Department of Medicine, King Abdulaziz University, Jeddah, Saudi Arabia
Adjunct Professor of Public Health, Ningxia Medical University, Yinchuan, P.R. China

Preface

The inspiration for this book came from the Spirituality Special Interest Group (SSIG) in the School of Human and Health Sciences at the University of Huddersfield. Members of the group were involved in researching and teaching about various aspects of spirituality. The concept of the book is rooted in the research findings and discussions we have had as a group. These focused not only on specific research areas but on the more general issue of how to promote a person-centred approach, with space for spirituality, in a health care system dominated by reductionist narratives of evidence-based practice, economic efficiency, and industrialised models of management and care.

We have dealt with the issue of evidence-based practice by addressing (and asking our authors to address) the considerable real evidence for the benefit of spirituality and spiritually competent care. We acknowledge that much of this evidence is based on qualitative rather than the traditional quantitative studies used as the basis of most evidence-based practice. We believe that qualitative methods are particularly effective in answering the 'why' questions about hope, meaning and the purpose of life that tend to be thrown up when we consider issues of spirituality. It also helps us to understand the lived experience of practitioners and patients alike. We have also focused on spiritually competent care rather than spending too long discussing the endless question of how to define spirituality. Spiritually competent practice is relatively easy to operationalise and we hope we have done that successfully, though far more research is still called for in this area.

The issues of models of management and care have also been addressed in various ways. We are convinced that fragmented and impersonal methods of care make it harder to practice with spiritual competence. Part of the task of good leaders and managers is to provide an environment in which staff feel valued and have time and space to provide good person-centred, spiritually competent care. Behind that there are deeper questions of political theory and the problems posed by austerity regimes.

We have tried to make this a book of practical use in promoting the development and provision of spiritually competent practice in health care. We have sought to examine the underlying issues and to make practical suggestions about how to tackle them. Many of our authors are associated with the SSIG but we have included a wide variety of expertise in our efforts to provide a book which is academically sound but also practically useful and spiritually challenging. We have enjoyed putting this work together in collaboration with our authors. We have learned from our authors and been gratified by the way in which people writing from very different personal and professional perspectives have produced a work which feels coherent and will, we hope, help us all to put spiritually competent care into practice.

John Wattis
Stephen Curran
Melanie Rogers

Editors

John Wattis

Visiting Professor, School of Human and Health Sciences, University of Huddersfield, Huddersfield, UK.

John has worked as a consultant in psychiatry for older people and in medical management. He has also coached and mentored doctors and others in management positions. He has developed his interest in spirituality in health care over many years. He delivered a keynote lecture on the topic of spirituality in old age at the International Psychogeriatric Association Meeting in Sydney in 1995. He has published on various aspects of old age psychiatry, and more recently concerning approaches to spirituality in health care. He is co-author, with Stephen Curran, of *Practical Psychiatry of Old Age,* now in its fifth edition, and of *Practical Management and Leadership for Doctors,* published by CRC Press/Taylor & Francis Group.

Stephen Curran

Visiting Professor, School of Human and Health Sciences, University of Huddersfield, Huddersfield, UK; Consultant in Old Age Psychiatry, South West Yorkshire Partnership NHS Foundation Trust, Wakefield, UK.

Stephen has many years' experience as a consultant in old age psychiatry with a special interest in biological and pharmacological aspects of psychiatry. He believes that an understanding of the biological, psychological and social evidence base must combined with good quality interpersonal care if we are to provide to provide the best possible standard of care. He is an experienced teacher and supervisor of psychiatrists in training. He has published research, books, chapters and educational papers on the psychiatry of old age. He has co-authored, with John Wattis, a chapter (Stories of living with loss: Spirituality and ageing) for *Spirituality and Narrative in Psychiatric Practice,* published by the Royal College of Psychiatrists in 2016.

Melanie Rogers

Senior Lecturer, School of Human and Health Sciences, University of Huddersfield, Huddersfield, UK; Advanced Nurse Practitioner (Primary Care) and Queen's Nurse, UK; Chair of the International Council of Nurses Nurse Practitioner/Advanced Practice Nurse Network.

Melanie has worked as an Advanced Nurse Practitioner in Primary Care and runs the MSc Advanced Nurse Practitioner course at the University of Huddersfield. She is passionate about holistic care and working with patients to offer hope during times of illness and crisis. She has promoted undergraduate and postgraduate teaching on spirituality in health care. Her PhD focused on spirituality in primary care and she has spoken internationally and nationally about this. She is a founding member of the Spirituality Special Interest Group at the University of Huddersfield and an executive committee member of the British Association for the Study of Spirituality. She was awarded the Queen's Nurse title in 2008 for her commitment to patient care and education.

Contributors

Gulnar Ali

School of Human and Health Sciences, The University of Huddersfield, Queensgate, Huddersfield, UK.

Gulnar has a particular interest in the ontological aspect of human phenomenon and her professional endeavours are keenly aimed towards human development. She has a wide range of teaching and research experience in mental health, medical anthropology and education. She is currently finalizing a PhD thesis on the integration of spiritual care aspects in undergraduate nurse education across England.

Laura Béres

Associate Professor, School of Social Work, King's University College at Western University, London, Canada.

Laura teaches and writes in the areas of narrative therapy and the integration of spirituality in professional practice.

Kevin Bond

Kevin has had a long and varied career mostly in public services. He has worked in many different areas of care, but predominantly in mental health. He has been involved in and responsible for several large psychiatric hospital closure and reprovision programmes and designed several national award-winning bespoke services alongside the people who use them. He was the lead designer and founding CEO of NAViGO CIC, a not-for-profit social enterprise designed specifically to run a statutory mental health service and associated social care, in which uniquely the membership consists of staff and people who use services and carers, all with equal voting rights. Kevin has also been involved with developmental work in other countries at the request of their governments. At present, among other areas, he is independent chair for a unique limited liability partnership of nine social enterprises across the north of England.

Mike Bush

Mike is Freelance Mental Health Consultant and University Visiting Lecturer. He has worked in the social and health care area for over 40 years. His experience has been predominantly in adult services and mental health, mainly working in Community Mental Health Teams as a Senior Mental Health Social Worker. He has also been active in social work, health service user involvement, and education for over 14 years. In particular he has been teaching sessions at universities in the Yorkshire region on the importance of understanding strategies to promote and protect the mental health of social workers and campaign on this nationally. He is a former member of the Professional Capabilities Framework Group at the College of Social Work, a member of BASW's Mental Health Education and Policy Group, and has provided training for BASW, Community Care Conferences and other social work agencies.

Mike Gartland

Michael is an Anglican priest and transpersonal psychotherapist working mainly in the NHS, leading a multi-faith mental health chaplaincy and counselling service in West Yorkshire. He has research and teaching interests in 14th century English mysticism and Buddhist psychology. He has extensive experience in leading retreats and of involvement in Buddhist-Christian dialogue.

Janice Jones

Senior Lecturer, Institute of Vocational Learning, School of Health and Social Care, London South Bank University

Janice has worked in higher education for 10 years. Her clinical experience as an occupational therapist is extensive and covers palliative care and end of life, patients with physical disabilities, long-term conditions and neurological impairment. Her research interests focus on how spirituality is embedded into the curriculum of pre-registration health and social care students, and the experiences of clinicians practicing with spiritual competency.

Penny Keith

Deputy Associate Director of Nursing, Quality and Patient Experience, Nottinghamshire Healthcare NHS Foundation Trust.

Penny graduated from Bristol University with a degree in theology and religious studies. Since then she has had a long career within health care including working as a District Nurse, Practice Nurse, Advanced Nurse Practitioner, and long-term conditions specialist.

Marilynne N Kirshbaum

Professor and Head of Nursing at Charles Darwin University, Northern Territory, Australia.

Marilynne's clinical and research experience is in cancer and palliative care, specifically in exploring how people who suffer with debilitating fatigue can summon up resources of vitality and energy.

Wilfred McSherry

Professor in Dignity of Care for Older People, School of Nursing and Midwifery, Faculty of Health Sciences, Staffordshire University, The Shrewsbury and Telford Hospital NHS Trust, UK; Part-Time Professor VID Specialized University (Haraldsplass Campus), Bergen, Norway.

Steven Michael

Steven joined the NHS, Wakefield, UK, in 1985, originally training as a registered nurse. Since then he has occupied a range of leadership and management roles in health care, including, most recently, Chief Executive of South West Yorkshire Partnership NHS FT (2007–2016). He gained an MBA from Sunderland University in 1996, and was awarded the OBE for services to health care in the 2014 Queen's Birthday Honours list.

Seamus Nash

Family Care Team Leader, Kirkwood Hospice, Huddersfield, UK; UKCP Registered Psychotherapist and Supervisor; full member of UKAHPP

Seamus is interested in the spiritual dimensions of health and social care work and the implications for practice.

Alison Rodriguez

Lecturer in Child and Family Health, Faculty of Medicine, University of Leeds, Leeds, UK.

Allison is a chartered psychologist with extensive teaching and research experience in health and critical health psychology. Her first degree is in Psychology and she has a Masters in Health Psychology, a Postgraduate Certificate in Higher Education and a PhD in Palliative Paediatric Care. Her work includes a focus on spirituality, self-management and legacy leaving. Alison uses phenomenological methods to explore meaning making and experiential well-being in Children and Young People (CYP) and their families.

Martin Seager

Consultant Clinical Psychologist, Adult Psychotherapist with the charity organisation 'Change, Grow, Live', Cambridge, UK.

Martin is a clinician, lecturer, author, campaigner, broadcaster and activist on mental health and male gender issues. He worked in the NHS for over 30 years and was head of psychological services in two large mental health Trusts. He has written widely primarily about mental health, male gender, compassion, attachment and homelessness. He is co-founder of a men's mental health research team running an annual male psychology conference at University College London. He has been a branch consultant psychologist with the Central London Samaritans since 2006 and is also a member of the Mental Health Advisory Board of the College of Medicine. He is also an adviser to the 'Self-Esteem Team' which provides mental health education and support to UK schools.

Jonathan Sharp

Spiritual Care Coordinator/Chaplain, Kirkwood Hospice, Huddersfield, UK.

Jonathan has worked for over a decade in the clinical chemistry departments of several Mersey Region hospitals, including Alder Hey Children's Hospital. After training at the Queen's Foundation and the University of Birmingham, he served 17 years as circuit minister in the Methodist Church in Northwich, Wakefield and Headingley, Leeds. He also served as a Trust Chaplain to Mid Yorkshire Hospitals NHS Trust for over 5 years.

Joanna Smith

Lecturer Children's Nursing, School of Healthcare, University of Leeds, Leeds, UK.

Joanna has worked in higher education for 15 years with extensive teaching and learning experiences. Her clinical experience, primarily caring for children with complex needs requiring surgery, informs her teaching and research. Her main research interests relate to the way in which health professionals work with and involve children and young people and their families in decisions about their care, in the context of children with long-term conditions.

Michael Snowden

Senior Lecturer in Counselling and Mentoring Studies, School of Human and Health Sciences, The University of Huddersfield, Queensgate, Huddersfield, UK.

Michael's research interests lie in the field of pedagogy, mentorship, curriculum enhancement and learning. He is a regular speaker at national and international conferences concerned with the development of pedagogical strategies. He is currently the national coordinator for the Flexible Pedagogy Group of the Universities Association for Life Long Learning and works in collaboration with the European Mentoring and Coaching Council to develop mentorship within higher education. He is a member of the editorial board for the *International Journal of Coaching and Mentoring.*

Phil Walters

Strategic Lead, Creative Minds, South West Yorkshire Partnership NHS Foundation Trust, Wakefield, UK.

Phil has worked in mental health for over 25 years, qualifying with a BSC diploma in Psychiatric Social Work at Manchester University in 1990. Creative Minds is in the process of becoming a Charitable Trust.

What Does Spirituality Mean for Patients, Practitioners and Health Care Organisations?

1

John Wattis, Stephen Curran and Melanie Rogers

'Why me?' asks the patient newly diagnosed with advanced cancer.
'What did they die for?' asks the mother of a soldier killed in the Afghan campaign, interviewed on the radio.
'How can I look after her at home without any support?' asks the husband of a woman being discharged from hospital with end-stage heart failure.
'How can I carry on?' asks the patient with severe depression.

Most of us will have heard questions like these in our daily work and sometimes from our friends and family. Where does the cancer patient find the *meaning* in what is happening to them?

How can bereaved people resolve their grief?

How can families cope when faced with the practical and emotional pressures of caring for their dying loved ones?

The answers are personal and they depend on many factors. Cancer sufferers may find strength from the compassion of those who care for them and even find personal meaning in facing suffering and death. The mother of the soldier, whilst sad that Afghanistan is still not stable and the Western intervention did not achieve all that it aimed for, nevertheless may have found some consolation in the fact that her son died for a purpose and for values that he and she both embraced. The husband of the woman with end-stage heart failure may find strength to cope from the kindness and practical help of friends, family and the community nursing/support team. The person with severe depression may initially need medication and even inpatient care if actively suicidal. In the recovery phase they may need to find hope and meaning through psychotherapy and connecting with other people. How people respond to such crises depends on their own starting points, their life circumstances and the support they receive from family, friends and professionals. This book is about how health and social care professionals can play their part in supporting patients and their relatives and carers as they face the challenge and distress of life-changing, sometimes life-threatening, illness.

The issues of *meaning, purpose, hope, connectedness* and *values* are at the core of our understanding of spirituality. Victor Frankl, an Austrian Jewish psychiatrist who survived three years in Nazi concentration camps, stressed the importance of the search for meaning in life (1). His pre-war work included successful initiatives in suicide prevention but he refined his ideas through observing how he and others dealt with the immense suffering in the concentration camps. According to Frankl, meaning could be found in three ways: through love, through dedication to a life's work, and through how one coped with unavoidable suffering. He developed a form of existential therapy which he called logotherapy (1). For him, existential issues were related to God and spirituality (2).

Spiritual Care Competencies

Van Leeuwen and Cusveller (3) reviewed the nursing literature to produce a list of spiritual care competencies for undergraduate education of nurses. This in-depth review defined six competencies in three domains. The competencies were backed up by illustrative vignettes and descriptions of key behaviours. In Box 1.1 we have adapted these competencies to apply to all health and social care practitioners and clustered them in the three domains (again adapted) identified by the original authors. We believe these can be a basis for identifying shared competencies needed by all practitioners.

Providing good spiritual care is part of whole-person, or holistic, care. Useful though spiritual competencies are in defining educational objectives, they are not enough. Holistic, or whole-person, care addresses physical, mental, emotional and spiritual needs and involves more than just 'possessing' competencies. It is not just about the competencies but *whether* and *how* we apply them in practice. This, in turn, is influenced by the work environment which can facilitate or obstruct practitioners in providing quality care. Holistic care demands a person-centred approach. We need to see the person using the service as a whole person with a life story, a sense of meaning and purpose, emotions and thoughts embedded

Box 1.1 Spiritual Care Competencies*

Spiritual self-awareness and use of self
1. Spiritual self-awareness and sensitivity to the needs of patients with different beliefs and values, and cultural and religious background.
2. Spiritual issues addressed with patients in a caring and culturally sensitive manner.

Spirituality in practice
3. Collection of information about spirituality and identification of spiritual needs.
4. Discussion with people using the service and relevant team about how spiritual care provision, planning and reporting are carried out.
5. Provision and evaluation of spiritual care with people using the service and team members.

Quality assurance and improvement
6. Contribution to quality assurance and improvement of spiritual care within the organization.

*Adapted from van Leeuwen R, Cusveller B. *Journal of Advanced Nursing.* 2004; 48 (3): 234–246.

in a matrix of relationships and shared beliefs. They are not just a problem to be fixed. Too often the focus on technical and economic issues (including restrictions on available time) makes it exceedingly difficult for practitioners to deliver care which supports the person in all aspects of their need. This is to the detriment not only of the service user but also can result in a demoralized, dispirited 'burnt out' workforce.

Spiritually Competent Practice

It is not easy to provide a good definition of spirituality. Later in this chapter we provide two examples, one brief and one meticulous in its detail. We could have provided many others from a variety of sources; however, we have found, as we have looked into this area, that it is much easier to *describe spiritually competent practice* than to define spirituality. This is the latest iteration of how we would describe it:

> Spiritually competent practice involves compassionate engagement with the whole person as a unique human being, in ways which will provide them with a sense of meaning and purpose, where appropriate connecting or reconnecting with a community where they experience a sense of well-being, addressing suffering and developing coping strategies to improve their quality of life. This includes the practitioner accepting a person's beliefs and values, whether they are religious in foundation or not, and practising with cultural competency.

This is based on a previously published description (4), in turn based on a description developed from observational research in occupational therapy by one of our colleagues and co-author of two chapters in this work, Janice Jones (Chapters 3 and 7). We originally modified the description to make it generally applicable to all health care disciplines. Later modifications include adding the adjective *compassionate* to emphasise the central role of compassion in spiritually competent practice.

We want to make an important distinction between *competencies* as the building blocks of what can be taught to students and assessed and *competent practice* which requires the presence of other factors to be fully realised. We can express this in the equation:

$$\text{Spiritually competent practice} = \text{Spiritual competencies} + (\text{Compassionate motivation \& commitment}) + \text{Opportunity}$$

Competencies have been discussed, and an idea of how these can be framed is given in Box 1.1. However, compassionate motivation and commitment in the practitioner is essential to apply these. This in turn can be supported or obstructed by the organisation, depending on how it treats its staff and whether it promotes systems of care that provide time for compassionate, committed, spiritually competent care.

Chapter 3 in this book takes a closer look at spiritually competent practice. Chapter 4 looks at how two practitioners conceptualise these issues and how spiritually competent practice relates to other concepts in health and social care.

Definitions of Spirituality and Religion and Their Limitations

Spirituality

Spirituality seems to be a 'tricky' or nebulous concept to define (5–7) and that is why we have chosen to focus instead on the more easily described area of spiritually competent practice. However, we do not want to duck the issue of defining spirituality completely. We first address it by looking at our own research into how health care educators define it. When, as part of a small study (8), a group of health care educators were asked to provide their own personal definitions of spirituality, several themes emerged:

- That self, person (or personhood) and being were central to understanding spirituality, both in the context of teaching and in the delivery of care.
- That spirituality gave a sense of direction, meaning and purpose to life.
- That spirituality (far from being 'other-worldly') was practical, affecting how people lived and acted towards other people and the outside world.

Spirituality was regarded as something that could not be seen or touched but nevertheless could be experienced. This led to a need to use different methods to teach about spirituality focused on experiential learning rather than traditional methods (8). This is discussed further in Chapter 5.

How do the issues our health care educators identified compare with conventional definitions, and how does spirituality in this context differ from religion? Hill and Pargament (9), having commented that religion and spirituality are related rather than independent concepts, characterise spirituality as the 'search for the sacred' but go on to assert that religion is also characterised by the same search. This reflects the North American tendency to see spirituality as less distinct from religion than is the case in the UK where Cook (10), after a careful examination of existing work, developed a definition which embraced both the secular and the sacred positions:

> Spirituality is a distinctive, potentially creative and universal dimension of human experience arising both within the inner subjective experience of individuals and within communities, social groups and traditions. It may be experienced as a relationship with that which is intimately 'inner', immanent and personal within the self and others, and/or as a relationship with that which is wholly 'other', transcendent and beyond the self. It is experienced as being of fundamental or ultimate importance and is thus concerned with meaning and purpose in life, truth and values (10).

This definition embraces personhood and relationship, sense of direction, meaning and purpose. To some extent, the emphasis on the fundamental nature of spirituality also accords with our respondents identifying it as being of practical importance and affecting how people live and act towards others. However, it is not necessarily a definition that can be easily operationalized or 'measured' for research purposes. In the end we return to the conclusion that it easier to accept, at the practice level, that spirituality is intensely individual. For that reason, it is preferable as already stated, to concentrate on spiritually competent practice in practical and educational terms.

Religion

What is religion? The Oxford Dictionaries online (11) gives the primary definition of religion as 'belief in … a superhuman controlling power, especially a personal God or gods'. Wattis and Curran (12), writing in a health care context, suggested that religion can be seen as a means of relating to God and our fellow human beings, connected with the beliefs and rituals found in many faiths and often associated with power structures; briefly, 'the politics of spirituality'. Some definitions would not necessarily refer to God and would implicitly include a number of systems ('isms') that we don't normally think of as religions (e.g. capitalism, socialism, communism, materialism, economism and even secularism). These may for some people function as a religion; see for example the critique of economism as a 'religion' by Richard Norgaard (13).

Psychologists have developed different ways of understanding religion. Allport (14) made a distinction between mature and immature religion, later conceptualised as intrinsic and extrinsic religion (15). Intrinsic religion is essentially religion that is 'of the heart', also described as 'religion as an end in itself'. Extrinsic religion is seen as 'skin deep', self-serving and essentially a means to an end. Intrinsic religion seems intuitively closer to what we mean by spirituality. Batson et al (16) added a third category to intrinsic and extrinsic religion: 'religion as quest'. This, too, overlaps with ideas about spirituality.

Secular Society, Religion and Spirituality

Most Western societies can be characterised as secular, in the sense that they lack consistent religious practice, belief or interest but generally tolerate diverse religious and cultural groups as part of the society. According to Stammers and Bullivant (17) these societies generate 'secular spiritualities' which make no reference to religion or ideas about God.

Secular*ism* is the term used to refer to philosophical and political doctrines that are reflected in the structures and procedures of institutions. One kind of secularism effectively excludes religion from the public arena and confines it to the private lives of individuals and groups. The other form of secularism, sometimes called 'ecumenical', advocates mutual tolerance between religious groupings and those of no particular religion (17). Nevertheless, there are boundaries that are often difficult to define but which can be crossed. This happened in the case of Caroline Petrie, a National Health Service (NHS) nurse who was suspended (but later reinstated) for offering to pray with a patient (18). It can be argued that the boundaries are not absolute but can be flexed by the mature practitioner sensitive to the patient's own spiritual position. It is interesting it was not Petrie's patient but another member of staff who complained when they heard about the offer. Boundaries also vary between cultures, with practitioners in North America generally being more willing to accept the idea of praying with patients.

The proportion of the population that are 'religious' (across a whole variety of different religions; predominantly Christian, Muslim, Hindu, Jewish and Buddhist in the UK and United States) is higher than many would imagine. It is around 79% in the UK and 84% in the United States (19). The number of fully observant members of their faith groups is much lower. Religion is not the same as spirituality or spiritual well-being, though for many people religion will be an expression of their spirituality and may help them achieve spiritual well-being. We have tried to illustrate the relationship between religion and spirituality in Figure 1.1. In its original meaning (see below) spirituality was considered as wholly contained within religion (Figure 1.1 a). In the post-modern era it seems possible to express spirituality and achieve spiritual well-being without adherence to a formal religion and to be an adherent to formal religion (at least in its 'extrinsic' form) without experiencing spirituality or spiritual well-being. This overlapping relationship between spirituality and religion is expressed in Figure 1.1b.

The term *spirituality* comes from the Latin *spiritus*, literally meaning 'breath'. The derivatives of the Latin root include words like *inspire* and *expire* (both used in literal and metaphorical senses) *respire* and, of course, *spirit* and *spirituality*. According to McGrath (20), the origins of the modern term *spirituality* in the English language can be traced to 17th century French. It originally denoted direct knowledge of the divine or supernatural. This would make spirituality almost synonymous with mysticism and place spirituality, in its original English sense, firmly within the bounds of religion (Figure 1.1a). However, over time, the concept has migrated so that spirituality can also denote an 'inner' life without any reference to religion, God or the supernatural (Figure 1.1b).

Harold Koenig and colleagues (21, pp.47–48) argue that in clinical practice it is often best to use the term spirituality rather than religion, precisely because it is so broad and all-encompassing. Swinton and Pattison (22), in the title of their paper, argue for a 'thin, vague and useful understanding of spirituality'. This approach enables the practitioner to start with broad enquiry and follow where the patient leads. However, for research purposes this vagueness and broadness makes it hard to distinguish spirituality and spiritual well-being from existential issues and psychological well-being. This issue is addressed in detail by Koenig et al in Chapter 2 of the *Handbook of Religion and Health* (21).

Despite the difficulties in measuring spirituality, there have been many attempts to do so. A systematic review by Monod et al (23) identified 35 instruments, classified into measures of general spirituality (N=22), spiritual well-being (N=5), spiritual coping (N=4) and spiritual needs (N=4). The instruments most frequently used in clinical research were the Functional Assessment of Chronic Illness Therapy — Spiritual Well-Being (FACIT-Sp) (24) and the Spiritual Well-Being Scale (SWBS; 25). Interestingly, both these scales contain subscales that relate to what might broadly be described as religious and existential dimensions. The SWBS specifically incorporates two separate scales for religious well-being (RWB) and

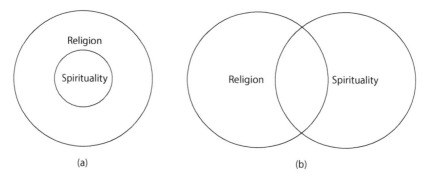

(a)   (b)

Figure 1.1 How religion and spirituality relate to each other. (a) Religion 'contains' spirituality. (b) Religion and spirituality overlap but are distinct.

existential well-being (EWB). When summated these give the overall SWBS score. The two components were designed to reflect 'two commonly recognised components of spirituality'. Items which score in a positive direction in both subscales certainly have face validity; for example, 'I believe that God loves me and cares about me' (RWB) and 'I feel that life is a positive experience' (EWB). The RWB scale (which relates to 'God' or 'a higher power' rather than a specific set of religious beliefs) tends to have a 'ceiling effect' in communities with strong religious beliefs.

There is also the complication that existential well-being appears to be closely related to what the positive psychology movement refers to as sustained or 'eudaimonic' well-being. This focuses on meaning and self-realization in contrast to hedonic well-being, which defines well-being in terms of short-term pleasure attainment and pain avoidance.

So, whilst the various scales may be good for specific research in specific groups, in the end we are thrown back on the realisation that spirituality is understood in different ways by different people. At the practical level, as Gordon et al (26) assert: 'The key to providing spiritual care is to understand what spirituality means to the person you are caring for' (p.5).

Spirituality and Different Worldviews

To fully comprehend the differences of understanding that exist, we need to take a look at different worldviews.

A worldview is a fundamental set of assumptions about the world in which we live, based on a 'controlling narrative' shared by people within a given culture. It acts as a lens through which we make sense of our experiences. Just as people are not conscious of the lenses in their eyeglasses as they read text, we are often not conscious of our worldview as we read the world around us. Nevertheless, our worldview alters our perceptions and can produce otherwise inexplicable conflicts between people of different worldviews. Radical theologian Walter Wink (27) asserted that there have only been a handful of religious/spiritual worldviews in history (see Figure 1.2). Wink described the 'Ancient' Worldview (Figure 1.2a). The narrative behind this worldview is that events on earth reflect events in the spiritual or heavenly realm. In this view, if two nations are fighting each other it reflects their spirits (or 'gods') fighting in heaven. The 'Spiritualist' Worldview (Figure 1.2b) is distinct from the modern-day spiritualist religion. The narrative here views the earthly, material realm as inferior to the heavenly spiritual realm. The material world is 'fallen' and true good can only be found on migration into the 'other-worldly' spiritual realm. The 'Materialist' Worldview (Figure 1.2c) became prominent at the time of the Enlightenment (mid-17th century) and is still powerful today. This view holds that there is no reality that cannot be reduced to purely material terms. The 'spiritual' simply does not exist, except perhaps as a psychological phenomenon explainable ultimately in terms of the physical world. The 'Theological' Worldview (Figure 1.2d) is a reaction to this, conceding the earthly, material realms to science and seeing the spiritual world as essentially separate or other worldly. This view is tartly criticised in the aphorism 'he is so heavenly-minded, he's no earthly use.' Finally, there is an 'Integral' Worldview, described by Wink as a 'new' worldview (though it, too, can be traced back to ancient times). This sees everything as having an inner (spiritual) and outward (material) aspect. We postulate that the integral worldview can be expanded into two variants, in one of

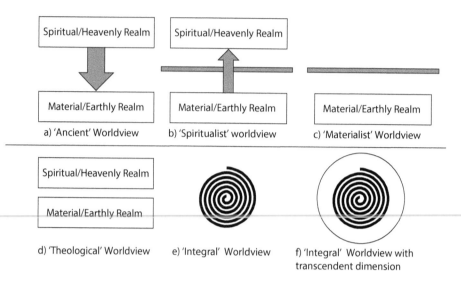

Figure 1.2 Different worldviews (27). The spirals represent an inner spiritual aspect and an outward material aspect.

which the whole of spirituality is associated with the material world (Figure 1.2e) and in one of which the existence of some kind of a transcendent, spiritual dimension beyond the material world is postulated (Figure 1.2f).

All of these worldviews and variants on them are still held by different people. Some are more powerful in one culture, some in another. Because these worldviews are largely unconscious, an individual's worldview may not be immediately obvious. Practitioners need to develop an understanding of their own underlying worldview and be sensitive to the potentially different worldviews of those they seek to help. To some extent our worldviews are culturally conditioned, but there will always be room for individual variation.

The Culture (Spirit) of Organisations

The focus on spiritually competent practice is one of the distinctive features of this text. The other theme that runs through the book is the importance of the organisational culture (what some might call the 'spirit' of the organisation) in facilitating or obstructing spiritually competent practice. Leadership is, amongst other things, about *inspiring* the organisation. In the armed forces people talk about *esprit de corps*, the shared spirit or morale of the service. Some see organisational spirituality as instrumental — a means to an end — as perhaps reflected, for example, in the title *The Handbook of Workplace Spirituality and Organisational Performance* (28). Karakas (29) conducted a detailed literature review on spirituality in organisations. He described problems in the workplace in defining spirituality (and distinguishing it from religion) similar to the issues we find in health and social care. Whilst recognising the inherent moral and ethical objections to treating spirituality as a means to an end, he nevertheless concluded that attention to spirituality could improve organisational performance. He summarised his review under three headings:

- A human resources perspective (improved well-being and quality of life)
- A philosophical (or existential) perspective (sense of purpose and meaning at work)
- An interpersonal perspective (sense of interconnectedness and community)

Again, there are striking similarities with our discussions on spirituality in healthcare. Certainly organisations can foster a healthy spirit of co-operation and common purpose.

We agree with Karakas that spirituality is more than a means to an end. For us, an organisation has a corporate existence and just as individual spirituality is concerned with meaning, purpose and values, so corporate or organisational spirituality is concerned with the meaning, purpose and values of the organisation. What is the organisation *for*? The declared purpose of healthcare organisations is usually concerned with improving the health of those they serve. However, neo-liberal political theorists have argued that public services were subject to producer capture (30). This, it was alleged, resulted in them being run in the interests of the staff rather than the people using the services. Competition was claimed to be more efficient. However, a privatised health system can end up being run for profit rather than for the benefit of patients. Compromises don't always work well, either. Handy (31, p.20) argued that the internal market in the British NHS, designed to deal with inefficiency and to open up the NHS to commercial providers, was artificial and substituted bureaucracy for choice (perhaps a different kind of producer capture). What should be the chief aim of health and social care organisations: profit, producer needs or providing health and social care? What should be their values? To most of us the answers seem self-evident.

More importantly still, where the organisation's stated purpose and values are different from its real purpose and values, a kind of organisational dishonesty arises because of incongruence between what an organisation says it is there for and what it is really there for. If the stated aim is to provide healthcare but the governing principle is really an easy life for the workers (producer capture — not that we have ever witnessed that in the UK NHS!) or return on investment for shareholders, the spirit of the organisation is twisted and inconsistent. An organisation with a healthy spirit is one that is focused on its main purpose in life. In the case of health and social care organisations this means providing care for people that is not only technically effective and efficient but also compassionate and attentive at the interpersonal level. If we look at the spiritual competency equation discussed earlier in this chapter, the organisation with a healthy spirit optimises the conditions for practitioners to provide fully competent care. In other words, the organisation represents the opportunity (or in some cases the lack of opportunity) in the equation.

Some would argue that many of the current problems faced by the NHS have been the result of excessive focus on finance rather than healthcare, a proposition supported by the findings of the Francis enquiry (32).

No healthcare organisation is perfect, but some do more than others to 'provide an environment in which clinical excellence can flourish'. This was the stated purpose of *clinical governance* (33) introduced to the English NHS by the then Chief Medical Officer Liam Donaldson in the late 1990s. Scally and Donaldson (33) emphasised that they saw a danger in financial matters and activity targets coming to dominate NHS

Board agendas at the expense of clinical care and believed *clinical governance* would be an antidote to this. They believed that financial control, service performance and clinical quality should be approached in an integrated way. However, finance and targets have tended to dominate the agenda. There are many reports of falling quality of care resulting, at least in part, from external political pressures pushing for an NHS governed by market forces (see, for example, Francis [32]). However, as Griffiths (30) pointed out, the market is not in itself a source of morality and social justice. The NHS or any other health or social care provider needs to have an ethical and moral code and a spirit with values that focus first on good healthcare.

Perhaps not surprisingly, clinical professions have codes of practice that put patient care first. The General Medical Council (34) asks doctors to 'make the care of your patient your first concern'. The Nursing and Midwifery Council (35) expects registrants to put the interests of people using or needing nursing or midwifery services first. The Health and Care Professions Council (36) expects registrants to act in the best interests of service users. The British Association of Social Workers' ethical standards also expect members to 'respect, uphold and defend' the physical, psychological, emotional and spiritual integrity and well-being of every person (37, p.8). However, when practitioners work in organisations that have double standards it is hard to maintain professional standards. When organisations claim to put service users first but really focus their attention primarily on the balance sheet (or meeting centrally set targets) they unintentionally put obstacles in the way of staff striving to realise their professional standards.

Obstacles like these are not unique to healthcare organisations. Stephen Covey opens his book, *The 8th Habit* (38) with a series of statements, including:

'I'm stressed out; everything's urgent.'
'I'm micromanaged and suffocating.'
'I'm beat up to get the numbers. The pressure to produce is unbelievable. I simply don't have the time or resources to do it all.'

This sounds like working in the health and social services. Yet this and other comments come from Covey's experience of people at work in many organisations around the world. He describes these employees as neither fulfilled nor excited but frustrated. He asserts that there is an eighth habit that adds an extra dimension to the areas discussed in his best-seller, *The 7 Habits of Highly Effective People* (39). Covey describes the eighth habit as 'the voice of the human spirit'. He defines the management problem simply: 'We live in a Knowledge Worker Age but operate our organisations in a controlling Industrial Age model that absolutely suppresses the release of human potential' (38, p.15). He characterises the management task as 'finding your voice and inspiring others to find theirs' (p.26). According to him, this is not a linear addition to the seven habits but as an extra dimension that cuts across the other seven. Covey believes that we need a paradigm shift so that people are not treated as cogs in some vast machine. The paradigm he proposes is a whole-person paradigm symbolised by a circle with three segments representing mind, heart (emotions) and body, with the human spirit in the centre. Spirituality is something which is integral to human functioning. It needs to be found and nurtured in ourselves and in other people. It is the antidote to the poison of mechanistic ideas of management.

Only a spiritually healthy organisation will create the conditions in which the human spirit of employees can flourish and reach their full potential. This will create opportunities to support the human spirit of people who use our services. One of the most important factors in providing spiritually competent care is the opportunity that the organisation offers (or fails to offer) to practitioners to make person-to-person contact with the people who use the services. Of course, resilient, spiritually competent practitioners will find ways to work around the system and be fully 'present' with the person, even when the organisation is dysfunctional. The self-care and organisational support which enables this is discussed in Chapter 6. How much better, however, if practitioners can work *with* the system rather than having to work *around* it or even *against* it to deliver spiritually competent care. In Chapters 11 and 12 we give two examples of organisations and projects that have, at least in part, created conditions that open the door to and encourage spiritually competent practice.

Different Ways of Knowing

Nomothetic Knowledge

In the context of providing healthcare with a spiritual dimension, John Swinton makes the very helpful distinction (based on Kant's philosophy) between *nomothetic* and *idiographic* knowledge (40). He describes nomothetic knowledge as knowledge gained by scientific methods such as experimentation and randomised controlled trials. This kind of knowledge is particularly valued in the materialist worldview and proceeds by developing and testing hypotheses. It is often concerned with *measurement*. According to Swinton, it has three key characteristics. It is *falsifiable*, *replicable* and *generalizable*. Knowledge is *falsifiable* only if it can be proved, at least in principle, to be untrue. A statement such as 'I love my dog' may be true, but it is not capable of absolute proof or disproof so does not belong in the nomothetic realm of knowledge. To be *replicable*, knowledge must be reproducible in situations other than the original experiment or clinical trial. Thus clinical trials are arranged on the basis that sufficient numbers of patients are enrolled in controlled circumstances to ensure that any differences between active drug and placebo are very unlikely to have arisen by chance. If a well-designed trial is repeated with a different group of patients with the same conditions, it is expected to replicate (yield similar results to) the original trial. Finally, nomothetic knowledge is *generalizable* to other populations with the same condition as those in the original studies. This kind of *empirical* knowledge figures strongly in the education of healthcare professionals and fits well with the notion of evidence-based practice.

Idiographic Knowledge

Idiographic knowledge is no less valid. It cannot be proved or disproved in the same way that nomothetic knowledge can be proved or disproved. It tends to be undervalued in the materialist worldview. However, it is open to rigorous scientific study mainly using qualitative rather than quantitative research. Qualitative studies are often concerned with *meaning*. As well as yielding results that cannot be found by quantitative enquiry, they sometimes enable hypotheses to be generated which are then open to a degree of verification using empirical methods.

How One Kind of Knowledge Can Lead to Another

Carl Rogers' classical research on psychotherapy provides a good example of how idiographic knowledge can lead to nomothetic knowledge. It is discussed here at some length because it is also relevant to how we teach and enact spiritually competent practice. Rogers' work initially depended on his detailed and honest exploration of what was happening as he worked as a child therapist. From reflection on these observations he described 'core conditions' of the therapeutic process (41), commonly summarised as follows:

Empathy — The therapist or counsellor understands the thoughts and feelings expressed by the client and communicates that understanding to the client.

Congruence — The therapist or counsellor is genuine and real in the relationship. This helps build trust in the relationship, and combined with the last of the core conditions it helps the client to have faith in their own perceptions and judgement.

Unconditional Positive Regard — The positive and non-judgemental attitude of the therapist or counsellor enables the client to speak about difficult areas without fear of criticism.

These conditions must also, at some level, be perceived by the client.

Rogers's core conditions have been verified by subsequent hypothesis-testing research over many years, summarised recently by Kirschenbaum and Jourdan (42). They also apply to human growth and personality development in the educational field. We believe they apply particularly to spiritually competent practice, supporting people in times of crisis, existential threat and ill health.

Preparing for Spiritually Competent Practice

Medical students and other health and social work students used to be encouraged to develop professional detachment to protect them against emotional exhaustion. This, coupled with the need to focus on the immense scientific and technical advances we have seen in the last 50 years or more, led to a curriculum that was unbalanced with too much focus on the more mechanical aspects of practice and not enough on the softer, interpersonal skills. Many older professionals learned their interpersonal skills from senior clinicians they worked with, in something akin to an apprenticeship model. More recently areas like communication skills have been incorporated into the curriculum but issues of spirituality and spiritual competency are only now creeping back onto an already over-crowded curriculum. In the United States, Puchalski has written extensively about and campaigned for spirituality in healthcare (especially medical) practice and education. Her work is summarized in her chapter Restorative Medicine (43) in the *Oxford Textbook of Spirituality in Healthcare*. Much of the impetus for these developments has come from practitioners working in end-of-life care like Puchalski, or geriatric medicine, where these issues are particularly pressing. There has also been input from the mental health field (44,45). In the UK, spirituality in nursing has been advanced especially by Wilf McSherry and colleagues (46–49).

Preparing students to practice competently in the area of spirituality involves much more than just teaching competencies. It involves different methods of learning. Respondents to Prentis et al (8) commented that there were areas where teaching on spirituality appeared to have particular relevance. These included specific subject areas such as oncology and palliative care and more general topic areas, for example morality and ethics. They also commented on how spirituality could be taught, including stressing the following:

- Encouraging self-awareness
- Reflective learning
- Sharing and modelling by the lecturer
- Empathy and compassion

Strategies for learning included discussion, sharing, narrative and poetry. When teaching about spiritually competent care, educators found themselves working in a more equal relationship with students. Indeed, a feeling of lack of expertise was one of the obstacles to teaching cited by respondents to the survey.

Respondents to the same survey suggested that the necessity to cover so may topics in education tended to push issues like spirituality out. Whilst around 90% of the respondents agreed or strongly agreed that spiritual values were relevant to their subject area and nearly half thought that spirituality was integral to teaching and learning, only 17% agreed that it was actually integrated into their curricula. There is still a long way to go, despite obvious progress in recent years. One respondent summarised it neatly: 'the time-intensive reflective methods of teaching needed in this area tended to be squeezed out in a performance-oriented culture that valued activity above developing skills of self-awareness and empathy' (8, p.49).

At the postgraduate level, spiritually competent practice can be encouraged and supported by discussion in the multidisciplinary team setting and through continuing professional development (often also conducted on an interdisciplinary basis) and by supervision, coaching and mentoring.

Chapter 5 of this book is devoted to how we can integrate spirituality into undergraduate and postgraduate education across the health professions (including those social workers who practice in the healthcare setting), and Chapter 6 looks more specifically at how organisations can support practitioners in caring for themselves and maintaining their own motivation and mental health when working in stressful situations.

Importance of the Personal Connection in Education

In their discussion of the role of the humanities in professional formation, Carlin et al (49) focus on the educational application of person-centred approaches. They report four characteristics based on the Rogerian core conditions that facilitate learning. The first is a perceived 'realness' (congruence) in the facilitator of learning. Then there is 'acceptance' or a non-possessive caring for and trust in the learner (unconditional positive regard). The effective teacher has to have empathy with the situation the students find themselves in (and to teach the students to have empathy with the situations patients find themselves in). Finally, the students must be able to perceive these conditions to be present in the facilitator.

Conclusion

The issues of *meaning, purpose, hope, connectedness* and *values* are at the core of our understanding of spirituality. In healthcare practice, whole-person care must include attention to spiritual issues. The concept of spiritually competent practice provides a more solid basis for practice, education and research than trying to tie down the nebulous concept of spirituality itself. Spiritual competencies can be defined for educational purposes but spiritually competent practice requires more than just the competencies. In addition, it requires compassionate motivation, commitment and opportunity. Motivation and commitment are usually strong in students and one of the tasks of education and continuing professional development is to nurture, sustain and strengthen that motivation and commitment. Healthcare systems and organisations need to be set up to facilitate opportunities for (and not obstruct) spiritually competent care. The distinction between religion and spirituality is important even though it is acknowledged that, for many people, they overlap and are integrated. The place of religion and spirituality in a secular, multicultural society needs to be negotiated. This involves understanding different worldviews concerning spirituality; being self-aware and recognizing that patients and colleagues may have different worldviews. Being explicit about these differences can help avoid misunderstandings.

Not enough attention has been paid to the culture (spirit) of organisations. Organisations that have stated aims in conflict with each other or with their behaviour create a spirit of confusion which can obstruct spiritually competent practice. Healthcare organisations must give the highest priority to delivering good holistic healthcare, and financial and other centrally imposed targets must never take precedence over patient care. Attention to spirituality in the workplace can enhance staff and patient well-being and enhance the sense of community in the workplace. Neglect of spirituality and a conflicted spirit can obstruct good practice and result in poor quality healthcare. The principles of clinical governance introduced into the NHS in the late 1990s support the same conclusions but have sadly not been implemented in a wholehearted way, perhaps because of repeated re-organisations and conflicted purposes.

A different but related form of organisational conflict results from current management practice often being too mechanistic and failing to provide opportunities for staff to truly fulfil their potential. We believe this over-directive kind of management is ineffectual in getting the best performance out of people and additionally tends to reduce opportunities for spiritual care. As Covey (38) stresses, we all need to find our spiritual voices and support and develop systems in which others can find their voices, too. Later in this book (Chapters 11 and 12) some of our authors show that this kind of development is possible.

Issues concerning worldview are also reflected in different kinds of 'knowing'. The materialistic worldview privileges a reductionist (nomothetic) kind of understanding where that which can be quantified or measured is valued above the other kind of knowledge (idiographic) which can be investigated using qualitative methods. Idiographic knowledge is fundamental to human relationships and sense of meaning. These different kinds of knowledge are summed up in the aphorism 'what counts can't be counted; but what can be counted doesn't (necessarily) count' (51, p.13).

Developing and sustaining spiritually competent practice depends on the kind of idiographic relational interpersonal knowledge that complements the kind of nomothetic knowledge, usually used as a basis for evidence-based practice. Idiographic knowledge can be just as valuable as nomothetic knowledge. This is demonstrated by the principles of empathy, unconditional positive regard and congruence derived from Rogers' qualitative reflections on his own therapy practice, subsequently confirmed using quantitative techniques and extended into other fields such as education.

Spiritual well-being overlaps with psychological well-being and spiritually competent practice overlaps with concepts like compassionate care and person-centred care. These overlaps will be further considered in later chapters, particularly Chapters 2 and 4. In Chapter 3 our authors develop more fully the understanding of what spiritually competent practice looks like. In Chapter 4 we have invited our authors to give examples of ways in which practitioners can exercise spiritually competent care. Chapter 5 examines educational aspects and Chapter 6 issues around how we support practitioners to maintain spiritual competency, particularly in less than ideal organisational environments. Then there are several practical chapters looking at how spiritually competent practice can be delivered in different healthcare settings. Throughout these chapters we have asked our authors to consider the quantitative and qualitative research evidence base but also, when appropriate, to include illustrative narratives. We finish with a chapter looking at how we might change healthcare education and delivery systems to better attend to the spiritual needs of practitioners and patients and how we might use research to improve the already extensive evidence base for good practice in this area.

References

1. Frankl V. *Man's Search for Meaning*. London: Rider Books; 2004.
2. Frankl V. *Man's Search for Ultimate Meaning*. London: Rider Books; 2011.
3. van Leeuwen R, Cusveller B. Nursing competencies for spiritual care. *Journal of Advanced Nursing*. 2004; 48(3):234–246.
4. Rogers M, Wattis J. Spirituality in nursing practice. *Nursing Standard*. 2015; 29:51–57.
5. Coyle J. Spirituality and health: towards a framework for exploring the relationship between spirituality and health. *Journal of Advanced Nursing*. 2002; 37(6):589–597.
6. D'Souza R. The importance of spirituality in medicine and its application to clinical practice. *The Medical Journal of Australia*. 2007; 186(Suppl 10):S57–S59.
7. Gilbert P. Breathing Space. *Community Care* 2006. Available at: http://www.communitycare.co.uk/2006/01/19/breathing-space-2 (accessed 30/8/16).
8. Prentis S, Rogers M, Wattis J, Jones J, Stephenson J. Healthcare lecturers' perceptions of spirituality in education. *Nursing Standard*. 2014; 29(3):44–52.
9. Hill P, Pargament K. Advances in the conceptualization of religion and spirituality. *American Psychologist*. 2003; 58(1):64–74.
10. Cook C. Addiction and spirituality. *Addiction*. 2004; 99(5):539–551.
11. Oxford Dictionaries online. Available at: http://www.oxforddictionaries.com/definition/english/religion (accessed 23/1/16).
12. Wattis J, Curran S. Spirituality and mental wellbeing in old age. *Geriatric Medicine*. 2006; 36(12):13–17.
13. Norgaard R. The Church of Economism and Its Discontents. Great Transition Initiative (December 2015). Available at: http://www.greattransition.org/publication/the-church-of-economism-and-its-discontents (accessed 30/8/16).
14. Allport GW. *The Individual and His Religion, a Psychological Interpretation*. New York: Macmillan; 1950.

15. Allport GW, Ross JM. Personal religious orientation and prejudice. *Journal of Personal and Social Psychology.* 1967; 5:432–443.

16. Batson CD, Schoenrade P, Ventis WI. *Religion and the Individual: A Social-Psychological Perspective.* Oxford: Oxford University Press; 1993.

17. Stammers T, Bullivant S. Secularism. In Cobb M, Puchalski C, Rumbold B (eds). *Oxford Textbook of Spirituality in Healthcare.* Oxford: Oxford University Press; 2012.

18. BBC News online. No action over prayer-row nurse. 2009. Available at: http://news.bbc.co.uk/1/hi/england/somerset/7873145.stm (accessed 21/12/15).

19. Pew Research Center. Religious composition by country in percentages. 2012. Available at: http://www.pewforum.org/2012/12/18/table-religious-composition-by-country-in-percentages/ (accessed 30/8/16).

20. McGrath AE. *Christian Theology: An Introduction* (5th edition). Chichester: Wiley-Blackwell; 2011, pp 108–109.

21. Koenig H, King DE, Carson VB. *Handbook of Religion and Health* (2nd edition). Oxford: Oxford University Press; 2012.

22. Swinton J, Pattison S. Moving beyond clarity: towards a thin, vague and useful understanding of spirituality in nursing care. *Nursing Philosophy.* 2010; 11(4):226–237.

23. Monod S, Brennan M, Rochat E, Martin E, Rochat S, Büla CJ. Instruments measuring spirituality in clinical research: a systematic review. *Journal of General Internal Medicine.* 2011; 26(11):1345–1357.

24. Peterman AH, Fitchett G, Brady MJ, Hernandez L, Cella D. Measuring spiritual well-being in people with cancer: the functional assessment of chronic illness therapy—Spiritual Well-being Scale (FACIT-Sp). *Annals of Behavioral Medicine.* 2002; 24(1):49–58.

25. Paloutzian RF, Ellison CW. Loneliness, spiritual well-being, and quality of life. In Peplau LA, Perlman D. (eds) *Loneliness: A Sourcebook of Current Theory, Research and Therapy.* New York; Wiley: 2012. Also available at Life Advance: http://lifeadvance.com/spiritual-well-being-scale.html (accessed 30/8/16).

26. Gordon T, Kelly E, Mitchell D. *Spiritual Care for Healthcare Professionals.* London: Radcliffe; 2011.

27. Wink W. *The Powers That Be.* New York: Doubleday; 1998.

28. Giacalone R, Jurkiewicz C. *The Handbook of Workplace Spirituality and Organisational Performance* (2nd edition). New York: M.E. Sharpe; 2010.

29. Karakas F. Spirituality and performance in organizations: a literature review. *Journal of Business Ethics,* 2010; 94(1):89–106.

30. Griffiths B. *Morality and the Market Place* (2nd edition). London: Hodder and Stoughton; 1989.

31. Handy C. *The Hungry Spirit.* London: Arrow (Random House group); 2002.

32. Francis R. *Report of the Mid Staffordshire NHS Foundation Trust Public Inquiry.* London: The Stationery Office; 2013.

33. Scally G. and Donaldson L. Clinical governance and the drive for quality improvement in the new NHS in England. *British Medical Journal.* 1998; 317:61.

34. General Medical Council. Good Medical Practice. 2013. Available at: http://www.gmc-uk.org/guidance/good_medical_practice.asp (accessed 30/8/16).

35. Nursing and Midwifery Council. The Code for nurses and midwives. 2015. Available at: http://www.nmc.org.uk/standards/code/read-the-code-online/#second (accessed 30/8/16).

36. Health and Care Professions Council. Standards of performance, conduct and ethics. 2008. Available at: http://www.hcpc-uk.org/publications/standards/index.asp?id=38 (accessed 30/8/16).

37. British Association of Social Workers. The code of ethics for social workers. 2012. Available at: http://cdn.basw.co.uk/upload/basw_95243-9.pdf (accessed 30/8/16).

38. Covey S. *The 8th Habit: From Effectiveness to Greatness.* London: Simon and Shuster; 2006.

39. Covey S. *The 7 Habits of Highly Effective People.* London: Simon and Shuster; 2004.

40. Swinton J. Healthcare spirituality: a question of knowledge. In Cobb M, Puchalski C, Rumbold B (eds). *Oxford Textbook of Spirituality in Healthcare*. Oxford: Oxford University Press; 2012.

41. Rogers C. A theory of therapy, personality and interpersonal relationships as developed in the client-centred framework. In Koch S (ed). *Psychology: A Study of a Science. Study 1, Volume 3: Formulations of the Person and the Social Context*. Columbus, Ohio: McGraw-Hill, 1959; pp 184–256.

42. Kirschenbaum H, Jourdan A. The current status of Carl Rogers and the person-centered approach. *Psychotherapy: Theory, Research, Practice, Training*. 2005; 42(1):37–51.

43. Puchalski C. Restorative medicine. In Cobb M, Puchalski C, Rumbold B (eds). *Oxford Textbook of Spirituality in Healthcare*. Oxford: Oxford University Press; 2012.

44. Cook C, Powell A, Sims A. *Spirituality in Psychiatry*. London: Royal College of Psychiatrists; 2010.

45. Cook C, Powell A, Sims A. *Spirituality and Narrative in Psychiatric Practice*. London: Royal College of Psychiatrists; 2016.

46. McSherry W. *Making Sense of Spirituality in Nursing and Health Care Practice an Interactive Approach* (2nd edition). London: Jessica Kingsley; 2006.

47. McSherry W. *The Meaning of Spirituality and Spiritual Care within Nursing and Health Care Practice*. Wiltshire: Quay Books; 2007.

48. McSherry W, Ross L (eds). *Spiritual Assessment in Health Care Practice*. Keswick: M&K; 2010.

49. McSherry W, Ross L. Nursing. In Cobb M, Puchalski C, Rumbold B (eds). *Oxford Textbook of Spirituality in Healthcare*. Oxford: Oxford University Press; 2012.

50. Carlin N, Cole T, Strobel H. Guidance from the humanities for professional formation. In Cobb M, Puchalski C, Rumbold B (eds). *Oxford Textbook of Spirituality in Healthcare*. Oxford: Oxford University Press; 2012.

51. Cameron WB. *Informal Sociology, A Casual Introduction to Sociological Thinking*. New York: Random House; 1967.

Spirituality in Western Multicultural Societies

2

Marilynne N Kirshbaum and Alison Rodriguez

Introduction

The societies of Europe and their close genealogical, linguistic and colonial descendants, countries whose dominant culture is derived from European culture, such as North and South America, Australia and New Zealand, are steadily increasing in diversity. There are forecasts that by 2050 there will be no ethnic or racial majority in the United States (1). Caucasian people may continue to dominate politically and economically in the Western world, but they will be defined as a minority alongside their ethnically diverse counterparts (1). The demographic profile of Europe's population is considerably more heterogeneous than ever. It was estimated in 2015 that Europe contained approximately 76 million international immigrants (2). The mixing of cultural norms brings both tensions and acceptances, and a merging of values.

Adapting to a new culture can be difficult for all concerned. Immigrants are faced with the challenge of learning about and adapting to new ways of being and communicating with others, attending to different social rules and trying to understand how services function, as it is likely that they will face many differences compared with their home country. Many adaptations can be stressful not least because of the demands on self and role confidence (3). It can be hard for people to adapt to new ways of life especially if there are conflicting ways of being. We need to consider also that these changes are often experienced alongside other life challenges and traumas such as loss and bereavement, especially for those seeking refuge or asylum, who have experienced war and rape, thus placing immigrants at a higher risk of experiencing poor mental health (4).

The aim of this chapter is to consider what the connection between culture and spirituality means for people living in Western multicultural societies and the implications of their belief systems for health and well-being. In exploring these phenomena we address the ways in which health and social care professionals can work effectively and compassionately with their culturally diverse service users and be more open to the spiritual aspects of their work.

Culture

Edward Tylor, an anthropologist in the 18th century, explained that culture is 'that complex whole which includes knowledge, belief, art, morals, laws, custom, and any other capabilities acquired by man as a member of society' (5, p.1). Over subsequent years there have been many more definitions of culture, each with similar key features (6):

- Commonality of ideas, meanings and values
- Social phenomenon, not inherited physiologically
- Patterns of behaviour influenced by common belief systems
- Belonging often at an unconscious level
- 'Lived experiences' modify ways of being and cultural perceptions

The most novel understanding is that culture can alter via lived experiences (7). We are not static beings; we may move our place of residence, become more educated and explore different types of employment. Our environment may also change beyond our control, for example, as a result of war or conflict. Even a governmental change can alter our outlooks, life experiences and expectations and as such bring about a cultural shift. It is useful to consider our own cultures as being in states of flux, be it at the individual or group level. This helps to prevent us from using fixed ways of trying to understand the cultures of others.

Culture and Spirituality

Regardless of our cultural origin or societal environment, we as human beings, as spiritual beings, psychologically connected to our worlds, are drawn to ponder: What is the purpose of life? Undoubtedly, the relationships we hold with ourselves and others impact upon our thoughts in trying to answer this question. Cultural expressions, norms and influences shape the meanings we attach to our perceptions of life and life's purpose. There are also instrumental factors that influence our worldviews, such as people and events, that make our lives not just liveable but fulfilling. Indeed, considering our purpose in life holds resonance in most philosophical writings and has direct association with spirituality. The mental processing involved in our perceiving of purpose gives us a sense of direction and a feeling of meaningfulness. Our spirituality however is not always something we can verbalise; it is instead often just a sense of connectedness to the world and its people.

Culture and spirituality are very much entwined concepts: 'It is often difficult to distinguish between the aspects of a belief system that arise from a sense of spirituality/religious affiliation and those that stem from ethnic/cultural heritage' (8, p.257).

Religion encourages people to think about spiritual issues in certain ways. People who belong to a religion and who identify with that religion's set of core beliefs can be and often are categorised by them.

Spirituality however, relates to an individual's meaning, hope and purpose. By the broadest definition, culture is shared and spirituality can be very individual in nature. For some people, their spirituality is highly correlated with their religion; their religion is also their culture. For others, albeit belonging to a number of cultures, be it related to race, ethnicity, location or work, their spirituality or spiritual needs may actually be in contrast to their culture's norms.

Spirituality and Personal Meaning

Part of the beauty of our spirituality is that it enables us to explore meanings and to appraise events from different viewpoints. We can live and story our lives from a number of perspectives. Indeed, many of us now in Western societies are at ease with stating that we are spiritual without being religious (9). This conceived postmodern phenomenon, or 'spiritual turn', for some appears to be making religiousness more private and individualistic. Spirituality is, as a result, becoming more valued as a vehicle in itself for supporting self-transcendence and personal growth; something that we can draw and reflect upon to improve our well-being and happiness.

Spirituality and culture undoubtedly structure human experience and our related values, behaviours and illness patterns. If we therefore view culture as a system of shared symbols and beliefs, then we can appreciate that our cultural landscapes influence our sense of being and belonging and provide us with the guidance for how to live our lives across the lifespan (10). For us to muse over the landscape of our spirituality in our Western multicultural societies, it feels important that we think about the rise of agency, away from historical and traditional cultural ways of being, and consider how some communities have been disbanded and how others have reformed with plural identities. Gilbert and Parkes (11) explored the place of religion, spirituality and mental health well-being in Birmingham, a large, multicultural and ethnically diverse city in the middle of England. The authors challenged the assumption of England as a secular society with this visual description of Birmingham as a city will observe a multitude of mosques, temples and churches that do not only serve as places of prayer, but are significant venues for community groups and activities. These physical spaces are intrinsic to a person's social identity and social anchors. Bauman (12) in his book Liquid Life makes a strong and relevant assertion of the importance of social anchors and warns that it is the disconnection and 'the loss of solidarity with other human beings' that perpetuates discrimination (12, p.11).

Others have agreed that a sense of spiritual and religious identity within a multicultural society can benefit all through embracing differences and helps us 'to invigorate the concept of the common good' (13, p.12) and react against the systematic dismantling of the anchors of social cohesion (14).

Traditional and Western Societies

Traditional societies with strong identities and culture will have behaviours that are prescribed and driven by a value system that has been passed down through the generations. In contrast, the values of our current and transforming modern Western multicultural societies are hazier. Our core values are less definitive and a point that we need to address in terms of health and well-being behaviour. Despite the general understanding of the impact of blurred values on our lifestyle and health behaviours, there is sparse empirical evidence in this area. Furthermore, it is a challenging area to research, as blurred yet complex values can be awkward to describe and measure. For example, they can be fluid, changing with context; they may also be deeply internalized, so deep that it can be difficult for us to even recognise or interpret (15).

Social philosophers and sociologists have written about the nature of modern day Western society and its cultural and spiritual implications. They stress individual autonomy and the 'I', or the self, as the centre of our world(s). We embrace our uniqueness, our freedom and choice. This postmodern way of being is celebratory and symbolic of the moving away from the constraints of the class system, religion and discriminatory practices. However, just as we realise with age that responsibilities are different and more difficult in reality to the notional, freedom itself can become a chore. We engage in the belief that our life is our fate and actually the choices we have, if any, are limited. This lonely road gives us little prescription. We can end up feeling that we have little guidance or ability to avoid problems that cause us to feel stressed by day to day challenges.

Following a review of the seminal literature and reflections on his own work, Eckersley (15) identified that despite our multiculturalism, materialism and individualism remain the main contributory characteristics of our Western culture. Materialism and individualism are drivers of our daily life. We work for heightened salaries; with increased monetary wealth we have the means to purchase more goods. This striving characteristic however has not bought us happiness. Increased wealth and possessions have been correlated with negative affect, including feelings of unhappiness and isolation (15). Materialism cannot provide us with our greater human needs of autonomy, safety and relatedness to and support from others. Therefore, if materialistic values become our ultimate goals, we end up living a life of disappointment. With increased material goals, we breed increased dissatisfaction with our lives, ourselves and others. Watson (16), using a sample of university students, found that materialism was related to 'shame', 'regret', 'low gratitude' and 'hubristic pride'. Things gradually become 'not enough' and our quality of life suffers (17).

In our striving for wealth, goods and possessions, in line with our materialistic selves and culture, we put ourselves at odds with what could be spiritual in our lives. We stifle our spiritual expression and openness to explore our spiritual sides. The freedom our modern Western culture has provided has distanced us from organised religion and regimented lifestyles, bringing us new opportunities for spiritual growth and development. But with this move away we have brought ourselves more worry, as we are not so united or in unison with others.

Spirituality and Behaviour

Our morals are instrumental to our religious identity. In a related sense, our cultural values guide our understanding of how we should morally conduct ourselves. Our knowledge of our own well-being coupled with Durkheim's (18) philosophies around social integration reveal that our societies provide value. Social responsibility and self-restraint are admired. We look negatively upon acts of anti-social behaviour and extreme self-indulgence. Our virtues and moral conduct help us to develop and maintain relationships, to be resilient and grow through difficult times. However, our individualistic and materialistic ways of being work against these universal values (15).

The impact of materialism and individualism is seen in the decline of mainstream Christianity. Cultural tensions have made it harder for people to include religion in their lives. As a result, we tolerate consumerism over religiosity, moving us away from seeking for the good in our lives. Still, if we consider all our nations, Americans have managed to keep hold of a strong sense of religiosity. However, other cultural clashes have brought about health changes that cannot be rescued by religious involvement. For example, America has seen a steady rise in suicide amongst younger populations. No correlation has been found between suicide and to what extent young people involve God in their lives, but there have been correlations found between suicide and measures linked to individualism, such as sense of freedom and internal locus of control (19). However, other cultural pressures mean that religion can no longer protect us from negative outcomes. In the West, we are more alone and our lives are more of an individual journey.

Cultures can evolve to erase the spiritual dimensions of their religions and replace those elements with things such as materialism, nationalism and fanaticism. Religion can still be instrumental in our lives despite this and can still offer support and meaning. Yet, the conflict arises when the traces of spirituality feel eradicated, the social value of religion then becomes too difficult to identify with because its transcendental nature is lost. Our desires for spirituality in our lives remain and there is an understanding that there is almost a current spiritual bridging of the old religions with the new. This is working to help us cope with the less spiritual forces that may be present in our cultures.

Spirituality in the Western World

Each person's spirituality is affected by their community and relationships. Spiritual well-being relates to how we feel engaged positively with others, ourselves and our environments. Traditional Western theories of spirituality and spiritual well-being are structured around the highly individualised self-concept. Geertz (20, p.48) provided an illuminating description of the Western world as

> … bounded, unique …[a] cognitive universe, a dynamic centre of awareness, emotion, judgement, and action organised into a distinctive whole and set contrastively both against other such wholes and against a social and natural background.

This perception of an individual who is bounded yet free is what Markus and Kitayama (21) conceive as the independent self. In a culture dominated by individualism – social customs, institutions and the media together promote the agentic way of being, pushing the notion of free will and individual reasoning. An individualistic culture supports individual efforts towards personal success. The dominant Christian religion in the West also influences this self-characterisation, suggesting that we are all created the same and personal rights are of the highest moral value.

In contrast to individualism, the Eastern view of the self exists as part of a collective. The self is not shaped by the individual and their unique needs. Instead, the self is viewed as being connected, fluid and flexibly bound to others. This is what Markus and Kitayama call the interdependent self (21). Social relationships are of greatest importance, not an individual's attributes. We therefore identify Eastern societies and cultures in terms of collectivism. Accordingly, many Eastern cultures focus on collective welfare and reward self-control, role performance and self-development in the more collective context.

These culturally entwined spiritual differences have implications for our shared conceptions of spirituality and spiritual well-being across cultures and within multicultural societies. Spiritual well-being is very much linked to personal roles and responsibilities amongst Westerners and within individualistic cultures. For example, we promote self-maintenance strategies (e.g. self enhancement), but interventions to enhance the individual self for example may be frowned upon according to some eastern philosophies. The need for positive self-regard in the Western sense of personal ability and achievement is not the most important concern of the Eastern or interdependent self. Instead fulfilment of role obligations in social relationships, the creation and maintenance of interpersonal harmony, the striving to promote welfare and prosperity of the collective (e.g. family) are central to life and well-being (22). The merging of cultures in the Western world provides us with opportunities to understand the other and to adopt other ways of being, to enhance our lives.

Health Care

Despite our acknowledgement of cultural differences, Western multicultural societies still operate within historically bound Western systems. The World Health Organisation's (WHO) definition of health, for example, makes no explicit reference to spirituality, despite acknowledging the impact of the social, physical and psychological. This perspective does not acknowledge that for some, spirit possession could be involved in some presenting cases of illness amongst ethnic minority individuals in the West.

Western health care is grounded in patient autonomy (23). It promotes individual determination, informed consent and disclosure of illness diagnosis/prognosis/processes of care to the patient as the ideal. Yet in many non-individualistic cultures family obligations take precedence, so there are spiritual conflicts. As an example of an Eastern, traditionally collective culture, Chinese family members are seen as a unit. The individual is seen as part of the whole so family members are always involved in important personal decisions such as medical decision-making; family members have a major say in anything involving the patient. This is because the moral philosophy and ideology of Chinese culture usually follows Confucian ethics. Autonomy is not a traditional part of Chinese culture and all the implications relating to decision-making are replaced by concepts and actions such as benevolence, compassion, filial piety, Jing (virtue) and Cheng (sincerity) (24). Filial piety is a well-established directive inherent in Chinese culture derived from Confucianism which infuses the qualities of respect, obedience and obligation into intergenerational behaviours. Children are required to look after and support their parents as they age and require physical, emotional and financial support (25). Similarly, in traditional Aboriginal communities in Australia, older people are protected to ensure harm does not come to them and will always have a relative close by (26).

Xu (27) drew on her personal experience of her father's long and debilitating illness to demonstrate how cultural differences can impact on health care experiences and spiritual needs. She argued that the notion of 'autonomy' had little relevance to Chinese culture and that disclosure/openness could cause harm. The Western practices of providing care and supportive communication, especially at times of 'bad news', neglected the collectivist cultural and spiritual needs of the family. Similarly, in their research on Japanese nurses, Konishi and Davis (28) suggested that the Western influence can strongly dominate all cultures as countries borrow Western advanced technologies. Along with this borrowing comes a

Western concept of ethics. However, trying to overlay one set of values onto another does not always work. The Japanese Eastern belief in the Taoism concept of 'non-action' for example does not corroborate with Western ethics. Amongst Japanese people, non-action can be a means of reaching spiritual enlightenment. In Western terms, however, 'non-action' would be in conflict with modern-day medicine driven only by action as a means to cure. In the West we deem it irresponsible and even unethical to not act or treat where there is hope for survival.

Despite the diversity of Western health professionals, they are educated to uphold the principles of autonomy and veracity. This is supported by professional standards and government legislation. The difficulty for health professionals in practice is when they are committed to conducting their practice within one set of ethical principles whilst caring for individuals from varied cultural backgrounds, each with different spiritual needs, values and beliefs.

The growing multicultural society presents health care providers with the difficult task of providing appropriate spiritual care for individuals who have different life experiences, beliefs, value systems, religions, languages and notions of health care. We observe that minority ethnic groups living in dominant Western societies do not acculturate to abide by Western ethical norms. They maintain their philosophical and spiritual values perpetuated through their cultural practices.

Growth and Happiness

In considering personal growth and happiness we naturally connect with the concept of subjective well-being which is associated with the positive psychology movement. Positive psychology concentrates on the elements of human behaviour that affect personal and community development. These are referred to as our universal character strengths and include the acts of integrity, forgiveness, kindness and gratitude (29). Suh's (22, p.63) metaphor of 'Self as the hyphen between culture and subjective well-being' is useful to aid our understanding of the construction of self, identity and happiness. In exploring how the self interacts with social institutions and people, we can begin to understand the meaning of spiritual well-being (happiness, life fulfilled) for individuals in different cultural systems. Contextual and cultural factors influence our spirituality and the manifestation of psychological well-being and so the patterns of expression of psychological well-being in various cultural contexts do need further clarification (30).

In studying subjective well-being, it is also relevant that we distinguish between happiness and life satisfaction. Happiness is considered an affective state that results from our feelings about life. Alternatively, life contentment is more cognitive and evaluative about life. Happiness is about feeling good, whereas life satisfaction is about considering how well we are doing (31). Our cognitions may convince us that with better jobs, income and wealth we are more satisfied with life, but this does not always correlate or show a direct relationship with us feeling happier (32). A few studies have explored the possible overlap in meaning and measurement of some constructs in the domain of positive psychology and spirituality. In these studies, the focus is to a great extent on the relatedness versus separateness of the hedonic (subjective well-being) and eudaimonic (meaningfulness) components of well-being (33). The hedonic perspective is focused on pleasure achievement, actively avoiding pain and discomfort, whereas the eudaimonic perspective is aligned with striving for the true self through the pursuit of goal-oriented experiences.

In contemporary literature we see many theorists drawing on the eudaimonic approach, for example in the work of Maslow and self-actualisation, Jung and his notion of individuation and archetypes and Allport's discussions of maturity. In drawing on these collective ideas we can see more clearly that the hedonic perspective of well-being is about having our individual needs and preferences met, which results in us feeling happy, relaxed and being free of difficulties. The eudaimonic perspective is more about experiencing the challenge for a wider, though still individual, purpose. This path might present the person with difficult situations and opportunities over the course of time, but will result in the growth and development of the self.

In considering well-being more widely, we know that in our modern-day Western multicultural societies, there are individualist and collective demands on our being and these can impact us in positive and negative ways. In terms of individualism, we account for personal responsibility, autonomy, freedom of choice, emotional independence and individual initiative. In terms of collectivism, we consider emotional dependence, duties, obligation and group solidarity (34). To achieve both, a sense of individual and collective well-being is needed to achieve our personal goals alongside the fulfilment of social roles for the 'collective good'. The extent to which our efforts are placed on our individual versus our collective well-being may be dictated by the cultures that surround us and the extent of our cultural belongingness to them. The individual will always have a choice, but their behaviour will be influenced in some way by the culture, rules and laws imposed by community and society.

A comparison of the perception of happiness was made between two groups of first-year sociology students. One group was based in Germany and represented a European individualistic, hedonistic and autonomous culture. The other group consisted of black South Africans and represented the collective culture of basing the extent of happiness on quality of close relationships with relevant others and harmony (35). According to this study, in the German culture group, happiness was described as being linear and incorporated an element of luck and the unexpected. In contrast, the black South African group viewed happiness as being non-linear and had attributes similar to Asian harmony and balance. They believed that having material possessions affected happiness. They were hopeful that unhappiness, affected by the lack of possessions, was temporary and would change as their status in life changed.

Karlin et al (36) compared the self-reported experiences of ageing in older adults across four countries: Italy, Thailand, Botswana and the United States. The authors were interested to determine what was important to older populations in terms of standard of life, particularly in the context of changing worldwide demographics. There were some interesting results. The elders in Italy mentioned healthy routines such as walking and visiting the senior centre. They criticised the bureaucratic process, which they felt was responsible for not having sufficient health benefits or funded services such as transportation, shopping, house cleaning and preparing meals. Fifty-two percent indicated that they were not happy. In Thailand older adults reported that they exercised and gardened, and just fewer than 85% responded that they had what they needed to be happy. The older adults in Botswana were the most active, suggesting that they had to be as they did not report receiving financial support from relatives, and government medical aid was limited. The US group had the highest level of happiness and health, participated in a full range of activities yet still needed more help with transportation, shopping, preparing meals and taking care of physical needs.

We have available to us a multitude of psychological theories and associated literature that categorises, hypothesises and explores our humanness. However, less attention is afforded to the social and cultural factors that interface between the individual and sociocultural elements of our being. Psychologists are showing increased interest in the experience of consciousness, and of spiritual techniques such as meditation and mindfulness as therapeutic interventions to improve our well-being (37). However, there remains scope to explore our spiritual connectedness with our cultural origins and developed selves. We are living in times where we are encouraged to seek out and adopt self-help approaches and to make sense of who we are and how we belong in regard to the past, present and future. In doing this we are thrown back to more indigenous worldviews (38).

Indigenous cultures throughout the world continue to strive to maintain their spiritual connectedness to their history, ancestors, land and belief systems through time-honoured practices, rituals and ceremonies. These cultures have struggled to exist and co-exist alongside the imposed constraints of modernity and capitalist governments. Meanwhile, just as yoga and meditation have been adopted into mainstream Western well-being culture, there has been a noted increase amongst non-indigenous people in learning about and participating in other spiritual practices such as shamanic journeying, moon ceremonies and fire circles which acknowledge and communicate with the spirit and metaphysical realms of existence. Although on the fringe of modern society, these trends represent a spiritual transformation located within the eudaimonic perspective. Some people are driven to search for their special truth, are thinking about making changes to improve their lives and are seeking out alternative types of spirituality and distancing themselves from the religious doctrines that they were born into (39).

The concept of *sukha* further contributes to our appreciation of different multicultural and spiritual perspectives that impact on well-being. Choudry and Vinayachandra (40) examined the different dimensions of *sukha* using the architectural analogy of 'space' and the symbiotic effects of the environment and the individual. *Sukha* literally means 'excellent space' in Sanskrit, which should be inclusive of internal and external aspects of life to which an individual is exposed. However, the word *sukha* is also shaped by cultural contexts, as the authors point out, since in India *sukha* refers to happiness, an individual construct. Here we observe another example of complexity in describing what is meant by happiness and subjective well-being.

Moving Forward: Cultural and Spiritual Competence in Health Care

Our current and likely future levels of diversity in the West have influenced our health care focus on cultural competence – from triage, to treatment and condition management. The concept of cultural competence and its necessity in the health care of diverse patients and families has flourished only within the last decade. Spirituality is also discussed as a concept alongside cultural competence, more so in the literature associated with death and dying and palliative care. Maybe this is because the anticipation of death and grief brings questions and desires that are more of a religious or spiritual content. However, increasingly we are seeing studies that are addressing cultural competence or spirituality in relation to the mental and physical health and well-being of all patient groups.

Research to date tells us that cultural competence is more than us gathering knowledge of cultural practices; it also necessitates that health professionals themselves consider their own constructs of bias and belief. Once these are acknowledged, health professionals almost need to engage in a bracketing out of themselves in order to provide compassionate care congruent with the needs of their patients (41). Cultural practices cannot be taken out of patient context and we therefore need to be careful that we are not guided by rigid stereotypes because we perceive a patient to be a member of a certain culture. It is what the patient believes, does or wants which should be what we translate into congruent actions. The modern view of cultural competence emphasises its fluidity: we need to be accepting of differences and understand that communication with patients and families is the main moderator in achieving compassionate care and potentially optimum health and well-being outcomes.

So what is our most important task?

Perhaps first and foremost it is to just listen, to afford the time to listen. We should also be focusing our education and practice around the concepts of personhood, dignity in care, good care tenor (positive attitude toward the patient) and compassion (42). Our practices need to develop with the aim of viewing our service users as people, each with hopes, dreams, wishes and desires. Rather than viewing service users in terms of just their condition or current health complication, we need, through our interactions with them, to show an appreciation of their cultures, contexts, spiritual needs and experiences. This way of thinking and doing should be mainstream culture in health care (43). However, health care professionals may be afraid to take this stance; conversations that explore personhood could draw too much on our compassionate reserves, could consume too much of our time, would be a real effort and could also be upsetting for the service users and health care professionals (44).

Many reports of patient and family dissatisfaction with care relate to health professionals not attending to their personhood with dignity. This is perhaps why health care, and especially medicine, is viewed as being distant and uncommunicative to the patient population. In her thesis (45), Rodriguez cites a number of parents who felt a lack of care and respect for personhood in consultations. One parent, for example, spoke about how she felt the presence of herself and her child was unimportant to the doctor and the nature of the consultation. She suggested that putting her child's heart on a petri dish would have been enough, as the child's physical condition was the doctor's only interest. He seemingly had no regard for the psycho-social implications of the discussions of treatment and intervention on the child and family.

Chochinov et al (42) recently conducted a study to test a time-efficient way of attending to the personhood of patients. They did this by asking the question 'What do I need to know about you as a person to give you the best care possible?' They labelled this question the Patient Dignity Question (PDQ). In this pioneering work, a total of 126 participants (66 patients and 60 family members) responded to the PDQ. The intervention was received extremely well by professionals, patients and families. Although generalisability of findings beyond palliative care is speculative, it is thought that this question could be posed to a multitude of patient groups and families from different cultural backgrounds. It is a means by which we can open up conversations about the person and their needs and from the outset make them feel that they matter.

Spirituality has been most explored as a nursing concept within palliative care, where related guidelines have been established (46). However, spiritual concerns have the potential to arise for people across all patient groups. Sometimes by focusing on the spiritual or cultural needs of the patient we can see that health and well-being can be assisted because what is needed relates to family issues and spiritual support rather than the physical needs of the patient (47). Mary Nathan in her Master's thesis, 'The Healing Power of Love', which was presented to the Royal College of Psychiatrists (48), explored the spiritual needs of psychiatric patients. She identified a number of patient needs that override condition and demographics. Attending to these elements of care should now be mainstream spiritual practice:

1. To feel safe and secure
2. To be treated with respect and dignity, facilitating a sense of belonging, of being valued and trusted
3. To have access to an environment for purposeful activity such as creative art, structured work and the enjoyment of nature
4. To be given time to express their thoughts and feelings to sympathetic and concerned practitioners
5. To have the opportunity to receive encouragement, to make sense of and derive meaning from their experiences, including their illness experiences

Being valued as a person can be enriching and there is a mutuality of care in this practice. Diverse spiritual/cultural needs can be acknowledged in practice, but we need to be inventive in our approaches, potentially construct new methodologies and languages (49) and consider how health care professionals are taught. We can work with the juxtapositions of cultural, philosophical and ethical values. For example, a patient may choose not to be told their diagnosis because of their cultural/spiritual beliefs. Witt Sherman (10) suggests that the best way to do this is to '… ask the patient whom the information should be given to and who should make decisions' (10, p.26). This way the patient is still making the primary decision – to receive the information or not. If health professionals conducted their care in this manner, then ethical conflicts could be avoided. Simply, the issue of truth telling becomes irrelevant in this context.

Health care interventions should focus on human flexibility and recognise the potential for complexity, regardless of the actual health condition. We need to be aware that even in difficult circumstances, people can devote themselves to the cultivation of activities which they perceive as challenging and enjoyable (eudaimonic). To this end, we need to consider:

- The development of models of care for individual optimal functioning – Are we attending to what matters?
- Exploring the use of methodologies that can sample subjective experience – We can learn from the experiences of our peers and service users.
- Evaluating both the objective and perceived effectiveness of the cultural environment and to what extent it fosters the Western value of autonomy and the integration of people with different values – Are we culturally and spiritually sensitive?
- Assessing family support to promote patients' independence, support and well-being – We can be more spiritually aware in our practice if we understand better the spiritual needs of people we serve.
- Developing intervention programs that promote patient well-being on the basis of their perceived needs and resources – This is more than a focus on cure or pharmacological intervention, it is about looking at the whole person.

A family-centred approach may be the most appropriate cross-culturally, as it aligns with collectivist traditions and is sensitive to structural differences in family roles and values. As the patient population in the West becomes increasingly multicultural, a body of evidence supports cross-cultural training, the use of cross-cultural principles and the appreciation of the needs of immigrant patients and families. However, research still lags behind real time. Some areas of study remain and include the need to explore further practitioner bias, results of cross-cultural training- and health care system handling of cultural practices that may bump into Western ways of service delivery (46).

Summary

We are living in an ever-changing multicultural world, full of people who hold and demonstrate different beliefs, values and behaviours. Even in times of peace, there are tensions and pressures arising from disparities of social, economic, psychological and physical conditions. It is within this context that a discourse on spirituality can contribute to greater cohesion and collective well-being through developing a measure of understanding.

In this chapter we have presented features of culture as a concept and explored how culture may influence our worldviews and identity, underpinned by spirituality, another closely entwined concept. The literature presents differentiating characteristics associated with traditional versus Western societies. Much of what we have found emphasised the collectivism of traditional cultures, often observable in Eastern and Asian societies, with the individualist and often materialistic priorities that dictate most Western, European and American ways of life.

Multicultural societies, where there is mix of cultures, ethnic groups, religions and spiritual beliefs, are heterogeneous and varied. We have included some empirical literature and selected examples that describe variations between people with different beliefs and behaviours. In discussing subjective well-being and happiness and developmental growth within positive psychology and spirituality, the eudaimonic and hedonistic perspectives were introduced, bringing more depth to the discussion with examples from different cultures.

The chapter concludes by bringing our attention to actual implications for the health care practitioner.

Conclusion

There is great potential for an exciting synergy of efforts that will influence positively cross-cultural spiritual care and the understanding of well-being and spirituality. At the same time, there remain a number of challenges to study the factors that influence the relationships between spiritual beliefs, societal values, concepts of health and illness, care and treatment. Most reported associations between culture, spirituality, health and well-being are correlational. We therefore cannot claim any direct causal relationships. However, the associations that are reported suggest that our modern-day Western culture does not promote our spirituality and is not good for our health and well-being.

Is this possibly why we are becoming more accepting of the new age philosophies and holistic therapies? Our modern-day drivers have perhaps made us lose sight of the precious nature of time, trust and togetherness, yet the pressures and negative effects have led us to yearn for the very same things (50). Still we return, from a multicultural perspective/worldview, to the universal imperative of human kindness and compassion.

Whether it is focused on the individual, collective, family or sub-group, it appears that it remains relevant and meaningful to us all.

References

1. Roberts S. In a generation, minorities may be the US majority. *New York Times*. August 14, 2008.
2. United Nations. Trends in international migration, 2015. Department of Economic and Social Affairs, Population Division. December 2015, No. 2015/4. Available at: http://www.un.org/en/development/desa/population/migration/publications/populationfacts/docs/MigrationPopFacts20154.pdf (accessed 6/16).
3. Rios PD. Migration and psychopathology. *Annuary of Clinical and Health Psychology*. 2008; 4:15–25.
4. Pumariego AJ, Roth E., Pumariego, JB. Mental health of immigrants and refugees. *Community Mental Health Journal* 2005; 41(5):581–597.
5. Tylor EB. *Primitive Culture: Researches into the Development of Mythology, Philosophy, Religion, Art and Custom.* Vol. 1. London: John Murray/Albemarle Street; 1871.
6. Institute of Medicine. *Board on Neuroscience and Behavioural Health. Speaking of Health Communication Strategies for Diverse Populations.* Washington DC: National Academic Press; 2002.
7. Garro L. Cultural, social and self-processes in narrating trouble experiences. In Mattingly C, Jensen U (eds). *Narrative and Society*. Holland: Reidel; 2001.
8. Miller MA. Culture, spirituality and women's health. *Journal of Obstetrics Gynaecology Neonatal Nursing*. 1995; 24:257–263.
9. Csof RM, Hood R, Keller B. *Deconversion*. Geoffingen: Vandenhoech & Ruprecht; 2009.
10. Witt Sherman P. 2006 Spirituality and culture as domains of quality palliative care. In La Porte Matzo M, Witt Sherman P (eds). *Palliative Care Nursing*. (2nd edition). New York: Springer; 2006.
11. Gilbert P, Parkes M. Faith in one city: exploring religion, spirituality and mental wellbeing in urban UK. *Ethnicity and Inequalities in Health and Social Care*. 2011; 4(1):16–27.
12. Bauman Z. *Liquid Life*. Cambridge, UK: Polity Press; 2005.
13. Sacks J. *The Home We Build Together*. London: Continuum; 2007.
14. Siddiqui SF. Islam and mental health. The 'Evil Eye' or the 'Discerning Eye'. 2009. *Conference by Birmingham Children's Hospital 30th April.* As cited by Gilbert P, Parkes M. Faith in one city: Exploring religion, spirituality and mental wellbeing in urban UK. *Ethnicity and Inequalities in Health and Social Care*. 2011; 4(1):16–27.
15. Eckersley R. Is modern Western culture a health hazard? *International Journal of Epidemiology*. 2006; 35:252–258.
16. Watson DC. Self-conscious emotions and materialism. *Imagination, Cognition & Personality*. 2015; 35(2):190–210.
17. Kasser T. Materialistic values and goals. *Annual Review of Psychology*. 2016; 67:489–514.
18. Durkheim E. *Suicide: a study in sociology*. London: Routledge and Kegan Paul; 1970.
19. Eckersley R, Dear K. Cultural correlates of youth suicide. *Social Science and Medicine*. 2002; 55:1891–1904.
20. Geertz C. On the nature of anthropological understanding. *American Scientist*. 1975; 63(1):47–53.
21. Markus HR, Kitayama S. The cultural psychology of personality. *Journal of Cross Cultural Psychology*. 1998; 29:63–87.
22. Suh E, Self M. the hyphen between culture and subjective wellbeing. In Diener E, Suh EM (eds). *Culture and Subjective Wellbeing*. Cambridge, MA: MIT Press; 2000.

23. Bowman K. What are the limits of bioethics in a culturally pluristic society? *The Journal of Law, Medicine and Ethics.* 2004; 32(4):664–669.

24. Tse C, Chong A, Fo S. Breaking bad news: a Chinese perspective. *Palliative Medicine.* 2001; 17(4):339–343.

25. Smith CS, Hung LC. The influence of eastern philosophy on elder care by Chinese Americans: attitudes toward long-term care. *Journal of Cultural Nursing.* 2012; 23:100–105.

26. Thompson S, van den Berg R, Smith K. The elderly: care and responsibilities. In Thachrah R, Scott K (eds). *Indigenous Australian Health and Cultures.* Frenchs Forest, New South Wales, Australia: Pearson Australia; 2011, pp. 152–189.

27. Xu Y. A Chinese perspective on autonomy (letter to editor). *Nursing Ethics.* 2004; 11(5):515–516.

28. Konishi E, Davis A. The teaching of nursing ethics in Japan. In Davis AJ, Tschudin V, deRaeve L (eds). *Essentials in Teaching and Learning in Nursing Ethics.* Edinburgh: Churchill Livingstone; 2006, pp. 251–260.

29. Peterson M, Webb D. Religion and spirituality in quality of life studies. *Applied Research in Quality of Life.* 2006; 1(1):107–116.

30. Keyes C. Promoting and protecting mental health as flourishing: a complementary strategy for improving national mental health. *American Psychologist.* 2007; 62(2):95–108.

31. Diener E, Tay L, Myers D. The religion paradox. If religion makes people happy, why are so many dropping out? *Journal of Personality and Social Psychology.* 2011; 101:1278–1290.

32. Lyer R, Muncy JA. Attitude toward consumption and subjective wellbeing. *The Journal of Consumer Affairs.* 2016; 48–67.

33. Ryan RM, Deci EL On happiness and human potentials: a review of research on hedonic and eudaimonic well-being. *Annual Review of Psychology.* 2001; 52:141–166.

34. Oyserman D, Coon HM, Kimmelmeier M. Rethinking individualism and collectivism: evaluation of theoretical assumptions and meta analyses. *Psychological Bulletin.* 2002; 128(1):3–72.

35. Pflug J. Folk theories of happiness: a cross-cultural comparison of conceptions of happiness in Germany and South Africa. *Social Indices Research.* 2009; 92:551–563.

36. Karlin N, Weil, J, Saratapun N, Pupanead S, Kgosidialwa K. Etic and emic perspectives on aging across four countries: Italy, Thailand, Botswana and the United States. *Ageing International.* 2014; 39:348–368.

37. Ecklund EH, Scheitle CP. Religion among academic scientists: distinctions, disciplines, and demographics. *Social Problems.* 2007; 54(2):289–307.

38. Coates J, Gray M, Hetherington T. An 'ecospiritual' perspective: finally a place for indigenous approaches. *British Journal of Social Work.* 2006; 36(3):381–399.

39. Ewing JP. *Reiki Shamanism.* Forres, Scotland: Findhorn Press; 2008.

40. Choudry A, Vinayachandra BK. Understanding happiness: the concept of sukha as 'excellent space'. *Psychological Studies.* 2015; 60(3):356–367.

41. Kumagai AK, Lypson ML. Beyond cultural competence: critical consciousness, social justice, and multicultural education. *Academic Medicine.* 2009; 84(6):782–787.

42. Chochinov HM. *Dignity Therapy: Final Words for Final Days.* New York, NY: Oxford University Press; 2012.

43. Thorn DH, Tirado MD, Woon TL, McBride MR. Development and evaluation of a cultural competency curriculum. *BMC Medical Education.* 2004; 6:38.

44. Meyer EC, Sellers DE, Browning DM, McGuffie K, Solomon MZ, Truog RD. Difficult conversations: improving communication skills and relational abilities in healthcare. *Paediatric Critical Care.* 2009; 10(3):352–359.

45. Rodriguez, A. We are here for a good time not a long time: being and caring for a child with a life limiting condition. Doctoral thesis. University of Huddersfield; 2009.

46. Kalish N. Evidence-based spiritual care: a literature review. *Current Opinion in Supportive and Palliative Care.* 2012; 6(2):242–246.

47. McKinlay EM. Within the circle of care: patient experiences of receiving palliative care. *Journal of Palliative Care.* 2001; 17(1):22.

48. Broster G. The Healing Power of Love. Research findings on patients' and nurses' perceptions and views on spiritual care in mental health practice and overcoming barriers to the provision of spiritual care: the place of compassion in clinical practice by Mary Nathan. Royal College of Psychiatrists Meeting, 8th November; 2001.

49. Tschudin V. Cultural and historical perspectives on nursing and ethics: listening to each other—report of the conference in Taipei, Taiwan, 19 May 2005, organised by ICNE and Nursing Ethics. *Nursing Ethics.* 2006; 13(3):304–322.

50. Harris R. *ACT Made Simple.* Oakland, CA: New Harbinger; 2009.

Spiritually Competent Practice in Health Care: What Is It and What Does It Look Like?

3

Janice Jones, Joanna Smith and Wilfred McSherry

Introduction

Embedding spirituality in health and social care is the essence of holistic, person-centred practice. However, the challenges and tensions involved in delivering spiritual care are well reported across health and social care literature (1,8). The very issues of defining spirituality and describing spiritual care are contentious. A consistent approach to developing spiritual competency in health and care professionals remains an issue. The quest for guidelines and models for the application of spirituality in practice continues; the absence of widely accepted guidelines continues to hamper efforts to embed spirituality in practice. At the same time, policy and professional codes of practice highlight the importance of practice that is holistic, person-centred and compassionate. This involves acknowledging the uniqueness of each individual and their experience of illness or disruption to their well-being (1–4).

Chapter 1 included a description of spiritually competent practice, based on the description derived from a concept analysis of spirituality in occupational therapy practice (5). This chapter builds on the concept analysis of spiritually competent practice. It draws on the current literature and recent empirical research in occupational therapy into how spirituality is embedded into practice (6). This chapter also addresses the issue of spiritually competent practice in relation to the experiences of patients. It examines professional experience and education and concludes with an overview of frameworks that might be useful to informing practice.

Background

Spirituality has been a growing concern for health and care practitioners for over two decades. The published literature available explores aspects of spiritual care from a variety of perspectives from diverse care settings. Despite this ever-expanding literature and evidence base, spirituality remains a contentious concept, difficult to operationalize in practice (5,12). The concept of spiritually competent practice has been considered by a range of disciplines, including medicine and psychiatry, nursing (7), social work (8) and chaplaincy (9). More recently the context of health and social care in the United Kingdom (UK) has been strongly influenced by high profile investigations into care which failed to measure up to professional values and failed to treat patients with dignity, respect and compassion (10,11). The outcome of these investigations has been to emphasise the need for professional practice that ensures patients are treated with dignity and respect across all settings, including respecting the diversity of patients' and carers' needs. One of the responses to these investigations was the National Health Service (NHS) England initiative to develop and roll out the *Culture of Compassionate Care*, summarised in the 6Cs of caring: care, compassion, competence, communication, courage and commitment (49). Embedding these constructs of person-centred care aims to improve patients' experience of care, well-being and quality of life. The initiative also requires managers to provide 'evidence-based' levels of staffing. The 6Cs can be related to elements of spirituality – namely, hope, meaning, purpose and compassion (5,12).

The intense media interest in these high profile reports (10,11), raised patients' and carers' concerns about their experiences and standards of care. As well as a political and managerial responses, a professional response was necessary to ensure staff had the attributes to deliver high quality care. These attributes include spiritual competence. The external barriers to providing spiritually competent care have remained consistent across the literature (4,6) – namely, time pressures, the environment and suitable locations to discuss deeply personal issues in private. Personal barriers potentially include the knowledge, skills and competence of the professionals. These are made worse by the lack of time devoted to spiritual care in professional education. There has been some progress during the last 20 years in describing and operationalising spiritually competent care but it is still not a routine part of everyday practice (4,13). For some professions, for example occupational therapy and social work, it has been argued that spirituality is integral to professional practice (6,8). In view of the challenging context in health and social care, developing a coherent framework for operationalising spirituality in practice is imperative for both patients and professionals. The following section explores spiritually competent practice, drawing on the literature from nursing, occupational therapy, social work and chaplaincy.

Spiritually Competent Practice

Spiritual support has been reported to improve outcomes for patients experiencing enduring illness, disability and in palliative care, for example by resulting in better adjustment to the illness (14,15). To effectively support patients' spiritual needs, the spiritual perspectives of both the patient and professional need to be understood; in some contexts clinicians find themselves more competent to address cultural issues than spiritual needs (16). The challenge is to realise these expectations in everyday practice.

The Association of Hospice and Palliative Care Chaplains' *Guidelines for Hospice and Palliative Care Chaplaincy* (2013) (17) recognise the importance of spiritual care as a core element of palliative care, and the expertise chaplains offer patients, carers, staff and volunteers in these settings.

The following sections explore the literature underpinning cultural and spiritual competency from patient and professional perspectives; we also draw on recent empirical narratives of how spiritually competent practice can be embedded in occupational therapy (6). The empirical narratives support a wider application across health and social care, emphasising that spirituality can be embedded into everyday encounters with patients, whether named and understood as spiritual care or not (18).

Cultural Competency

Culture has been described as the shared experiences and way of life impacting on an individual's attitudes and behaviour and shaped by early formative experiences and choices (8,19). Cultural competency has been defined as 'a set of congruent behaviours, attitudes and policies that come together in a system or agency or among professionals that enables effective work in cross cultural situations' (19, p.623).

In social work practice, cultural competence has been inextricably linked to race, ethnicity and spirituality; it has been described as the lens through which the individual's worldview, beliefs, values and norms are viewed and shared (20).

For many professionals the terms spirituality and religiosity (used in the non-pejorative sense) have been considered interchangeable despite their conceptual differences (21). Spiritual competence has been linked to cultural competence in the outworking of sensitivity to patients' culturally influenced characteristics. Spiritual competency has been considered a more focused expression of cultural competency, with professional competence attributed to the knowledge, skills and attitudes portrayed by an individual practitioner (20). The application of spiritual and cultural competency to practice demonstrates the inextricable links between them. Health and social care professionals need to appreciate the underpinning constructs of an individual's culture, determining who they are and their wish to be treated with dignity and respect. By understanding these cultural aspects the professional is equipped to explore and understand the unique spiritual constructs essential to a patient's life, care and experience of illness. Failing to embed these constructs leads to a failure in the provision of holistic care (20,21).

Meeting the needs of a diverse population is demanding. The demographic changes in the population of the UK (and globally) over the past 20 years have demanded an increased professional awareness of different cultures, their understanding of health and well-being and patient expectations. At the same time there has been a trend towards a more secular society, which has also impacted on health and social care practice. Between 2001 and 2011 the number of people identifying themselves as Christian reduced from 72% to 59%, with those identifying as having no religion accounting for 25% of the population in 2011 (22). A more recent survey in 2014 has shown 48.5% identifying as no religion with only 25% identifying as Christian (23).

The process of developing cultural competence is dynamic. Cultural competence demands a willingness for professionals to develop an awareness and acceptance of cultural diversity, acquiring knowledge of cultural differences and similarities. An awareness and self examination of one's own cultural values and identity, the development of lifelong learning and reflective practice facilitate the adaptation of skills and services to diverse cultures. Underpinning these attributes is the requirement for effective communication across cultural groups encountered in practice (19).

Components of Spiritually Competent Practice

Spiritual competency is an integral expression and manifestation of cultural competence. It is a dynamic and developmental process developed through an integration of attitudes, knowledge and skills developed over time. Spiritually competent practice can be characterised by three interrelated dimensions:

1. Knowledge of personal worldview
2. Empathetic appreciation of other worldviews different from one's own
3. The ability to develop strategies and interventions that reflect an individual's worldview and cultural perspective (20)

Despite much being written about the need for health and care professions to deliver spiritually competent care, it remains problematic. This has been attributed in part to professional insecurity and an uncertainty about the how to embed spiritually in everyday care (24). An increased focus on spiritual care is needed across both pre-and post-registration education as an essential precursor to developing spiritually competent care in practice (25).

A strong indicator for health and social care professionals' ability to provide spiritual care is the individual's understanding and awareness of their own spirituality. An understanding of their own personal beliefs and biases and how these impact on care delivery provides a lens through which they view their practice. This self-awareness supports the empathetic development and understanding of other people's spiritual needs (5,6,26).

One problematic area is applying spirituality in practice (28). The assessment and implementation of spiritual care has been cited as the most difficult area for student nurses (26,27). The Royal College of Nursing survey (29), investigating nurses' perceptions of spirituality and spiritual care, highlighted the following areas nurses considered to be spiritual care:

- Supporting the patient who is suffering
- Compassionate care; respecting the dignity of the patient in nursing procedures and care practices
- Communication; giving patients time to express themselves, and listening to them
- Being present (or being with) at a time of spiritual need, adopting a relaxed style

Ultimately nurses described their practice in terms of the qualities, behaviours and skills necessary to provide spiritually competent nursing practice, despite reporting they lacked competence in spiritual care. Nurses consistently reported lacking the educational preparation to address spirituality in practice. That lack of knowledge made them uncertain and unprepared to address the spiritual needs of patents, hindering spiritually competent practice.

Occupational Therapy Practice

A concept analysis of how occupational therapists address spirituality found that occupational therapy practice included elements of spirituality at the level of delivering care interventions (6). The historical roots of occupational therapy and nursing both include spirituality as a core construct of holistic practice, central to the philosophy of the professions (6,30). However, as health care practice sought to use science as the ultimate focus, occupational therapy developed a more reductionist approach and drifted from its founding philosophies and principles (6). More recently, the reawakening of the core philosophy of the profession has been evident, and a number of researchers have explored what the spiritual dimension of holistic practice looks like for occupational therapists (6).

Spirituality is recognised as a core domain of occupational therapy practice, although it is difficult to find evidence of a coherent definition to support putting the concept into practice (5,28). A concept analysis undertaken by Jones et al (5) identified the antecedents, defining attributes and consequences of spiritual care in occupational therapy practice, and offered a framework for practice. Table 3.1 shows how the antecedents, defining attributes and consequences of spirituality in occupational therapy practice were framed.

Table 3.1 Antecedents, Defining Attributes and Consequences of Spirituality in Occupational Therapy Practice

Antecedents	Defining Attributes	Consequences
Disruption to a person's health status affecting their well-being and quality of life; for example: • Acute illness • Mental health problem • Terminal diagnosis • End of life • Loss or grief	Addressing suffering related to the individual's circumstances; the provision of a holistic, person-centred approach to occupational therapy practice; the therapeutic relationship facilitates addressing a patient's spiritual needs	Individuals' experience well-being through a sense of meaning and purpose in their life and spiritual order, and work towards the restoration of values and a belief system
Disruption may lead to: • Loss of 'flow' in a person's occupations and life balance • Loss of 'meaning' and 'purpose', and 'significance' in life • Loss of purpose in life with the consequence of lowered self esteem • Lack of 'values' in life • Lack of connection within life • Lack of ability to transcend disruptions	Attributes of disruption reflected the dimensions of PSI framework (56): Becoming Meaning Being Centeredness Connectedness Transcendence	Recognition of inner resources assists coping with disruptive situations in a person's life, either temporary or permanent Spiritual order exists when an individual can reconcile most or all PSI dimensions of spirituality (56)

Source: Jones J, Topping A, Wattis J, Smith J., *Journal for the Study of Spirituality.* 2016; (6)1:38–57. Copyright British Association for the Study of Spirituality and Maney, reprinted by permission of Taylor & Francis Group (www.tandfonline.com) on behalf of British Association for the Study of Spirituality and Maney.

The findings from the concept analysis were mapped to the psychospiritual frame of reference for occupational therapy (31). These are characterised as *becoming, meaning, being, centeredness, connectedness* and *transcendence* with an additional construct *suffering*, added to reflect the literature (31,32). These spiritual constructs and their relevance to embedding spirituality into contemporary occupational therapy practice are discussed below. The themes are relevant and can be applied widely to all health and social care professionals. Quotes are from interviews with a number of occupational therapists interviewed in a PhD study (6).

Meaning: Refers to exploring the meaning associated with illness or disability; establishing meaningful pursuits and goals which enhance quality of life and well-being (5,32). An example of how occupational therapists facilitate the experiences of meaning and purpose in patient's lives is outlined in the following account:

> ... she was on empty ... manifesting in her symptoms [fatigue and anxiety] so I was trying to think of things that I tried a variety of methods to get her to look at what she loved. To put that into her life and give her that joy and hope ... it sounds really simple I just find that write down things that cost nothing like watching the rain running down the window ... looking at blossom on the tree outside ... that was a breakthrough moment for her ... Fatigue management isn't about managing fatigue it's actually changing your way of life that brings you meaning and purpose (6, pp.156–157).

Connectedness: Refers to the experience of belonging to others, God, nature and family, facilitated in practice by supporting connections with communities and spiritual practices. Connections are strengthened by the patient–therapist relationship supporting the facilitation of therapeutic interventions (5,31,32).The following account illustrates how the connection between the patient and therapist, and the therapeutic relationship were important when delivering bad news:

> ... I think back to the gentleman who was never going to walk again and you know ... it was a real challenge to kind of find the place, find the words, set the environment up; without just coming out and doing ... saying you know ... you're not going to walk again ... whereas building that therapeutic relationship, using the best environment and articulating that in, in a functional perspective and actually looking at, you know, whilst this is the case ... it goes back to the whole thing of hope ... looking about kind of ... that is catastrophic (6, p.156).

Transcendence: Can be described as the capacity to look beyond the immediate environment and draw on existential feelings of power or forces beyond the individual. Developing the capacity to change behaviours and strategies to cope with illness or disruptive situations requiring existential resources is a creature of transcendence. Notably, an application of transcendence is evident when facilitating coping strategies or end of life discussions, and closely linked to meaning and purpose. Relaxation, anxiety management, dealing with loss and grief are further examples of the application of transcendence to practice (5,31,32). Engaging in spiritually uplifting occupations such as gardening provides a patient with connections to resources beyond their internal control as highlighted in the following account:

> Spirituality is ingrained in occupation. I'm thinking of the patient who just said that he connected with something bigger than himself when he was out in the garden in the open air. You know that's

sometimes described as a higher power. To me that's, oh so spiritual you know that he connected to God with doing something outside (6, p.162).

Becoming: Refers to the individual's personal capacity for growth and change, and the potential to achieve self-actualisation. The following interventions focus on *becoming*: promoting autonomy, independence, facilitating choice and adaptation to illness or disability. For example, self-healing activities such as worship, relaxation, stress management and improving social and life skills all promote the spiritual dimension of becoming (32). The account below illustrates how occupational therapy interventions can be effective helping a patient to realise their potential in the face of disruption:

> I remember going to see a patient to see how she could get her tights on. The patient had a progressive neurological condition and was deteriorating. Her roles had really taken a knock and she was no longer working as a teacher. But she's really funky in her dress and she goes to vintage fairs and she'd found some Mary Quant tights. ... It was, um, for her being able to put on a pair of tights she wanted and do it independently was so big, and would make her feel really good about herself. Just a small thing but the essence of what we do (6, p.160).

Being: Can be described as the essence of the person, the individual characteristics that make a person unique, therefore the embodiment of person-centred practice. Application of *being* to practice can be appreciated in the personal skills of the therapist to embed person-centred practice such as listening skills, acknowledging the individual's beliefs and values. Facilitating the time and space to discuss spiritual or religious concerns, values, desires and dreams (5,31,32). How an occupational therapist works with an individual patient embedding person-centred care and acknowledging the uniqueness of their experiences and situation, is highlighted below:

> I think, I am aware that everyone's an individual, everyone has individualistic needs. ... I think I just do what I ... I do what I do, and I take cues from obviously the individual and their relatives ... and trying to appreciate what they are going through. Trying to see things from their point of view, look at the impact it would have on their lives and roles in the future ... try to empathise with how they are feeling. You know, about what I'm suggesting or changes that need to be made ... and the reason why that would be the case. But try to work with them at the same time (6, p.154).

Centeredness: Describes the acknowledgement of an individual's spirituality and/or religious expression linked to the notion of achieving spiritual well-being through activities such as meditation or creative visualisation. The purpose of these activities is to create a balance in a person's life where the chaotic factors from illness or grief have disrupted their sense of well-being. Centeredness promotes the opportunity for facilitating religious or spiritual practices, such as attending worship. Thus the domain of centeredness and connection are interlinked (5,31). The following extract from observation fieldwork notes illustrates how occupational therapists intervene in situations where grief has impacted on a patient's well-being in order to facilitate the patient's sense of control in the context of disruptive factors:

The occupational therapist was discussing the multiple losses that the patient had experienced recently. The patient talked about her recent surgery to remove a brain tumour, the loss of her job and car as a result of her illnesses. She had also just lost her mother and the recent funeral was discussed, exploring how the patient was feeling. Her resulting anxiety and grief from these multiple losses was acknowledged and the patient reassured that grief and anxiety in all its forms can have an impact on fatigue. The occupational therapist reflected to the patient how this affected her [the patient's] spirit saying, 'This all affects you deep down in your spirit' (6, p.155).

Suffering: The construct of suffering, in relation to spirituality, is an essential aspect of our humanity (33). The pressures of modern health care make it a challenge to provide a context where a patient can experience a supportive and life-sustaining environment as they experience pain and suffering (34). Martinson suggests hospital environments should be places where patients can 'dwell', with the notion of safety, support and a sense of belonging which goes beyond the adherence to satisfying a patient's needs and working to protocols. Suffering is supported in practice by empathising with the person's pain and/ or loss before progressing to practical interventions and therapy (32). The following account highlights how empathising with suffering from pain and lack of sleep led to addressing the patient's difficulties by providing equipment:

> You know in terms of somebody's sort of condition and being at the end of their life, you know, in terms of their sort of functional ability and being impaired, um, I've sometimes found that it is the smallest of things that have made such a big difference to people and like the gentleman we saw about the sleep system. He cannot sort of actively engage in any tasks now. But having the sleep system prevented pain and discomfort. And made him, knowing he could sleep aligned, psychologically made him feel better. … I think it's giving him a sense of comfort and safety … cause having a good night's sleep has a massive impact on the next day, doesn't it? (6, p.159)

In the absence of a congruent definition which describes spiritually, the description below is offered as a means of increasing the occupational therapist's understanding of how spirituality can be applied coherently in practice (5, p.16):

> Spiritually competent occupational therapy practice engages a person, as a unique spiritual being, in occupations which will provide them with a sense of meaning and purpose. It seeks to connect or reconnect them with a community where they experience a sense of well-being, addresses suffering and develops coping strategies to improve their quality of life. This includes the occupational therapist accepting a person's belief and values whether they are religious in foundation or not and practicing with cultural competency (5).

This description of spiritually competent practice, derived from occupational therapy research, has portability to other health and social care professions. Earlier, in Chapter 1, the authors have used this description to devise a description which is more broadly applicable across health and social care professions.

In contrast to the concept analysis (5) based solely on empirical literature from occupational therapy practice, Weathers et al (12) focused their analysis on empirical and conceptual literature from a wide range of health care professions including nursing, allied health, medicine, psychology, pastoral care, education, theology and social work. Their defining attributes (connectedness, transcendence and meaning in life) relate to the findings in the occupational therapy literature. However, the antecedents focus more broadly on the spiritual experience such as belief system and/or philosophical worldview. Both studies suggested that difficult life events such as illness or disruptions to well-being were antecedents for spiritual need to occur. The consequences in both studies focus on the individual's ability to develop coping strategies that enhance quality of life and well-being. Both studies suggest a commonality about the elements understood to frame spirituality and support our understanding of the constructs of spiritually competent practice.

Patients' Experiences of Spiritually Competent Care

Whilst there is an abundance of literature on spirituality and the experiences of health and care professionals, there is a paucity of research exploring the impact of spiritually competent care on patients. The contemporary context of patient care in the UK is influenced by the sociological and economic factors common to many developed countries. Demographically, there is an ageing population with an elderly population living longer with increased disability, placing additional strain on finite resources and services. Economically the NHS has recently faced austerity measures affecting care delivery. Services have faced demands for increased efficiency and throughput of patients with increasing financial constraints. The observational study, as previously outlined (6), identified the organisation and contextual challenges to occupational therapists embedding spirituality in practice as

- Time restraints leading to limited interventions (rushed care)
- Organizational targets to increase the throughput of patients (target-driven interventions)
- Pressure to adhere to bed management strategies

These pressures were effectively managed by a resilient and experienced sample of occupational therapists. Their practice context and the experience of the patient were at variance with practitioners' core professional philosophies and values. They were charged with practising in a context where the conflicts between policy, the reality of service delivery and professional values created additional stresses (6).

Studies exploring the experiences of patients and carers suggest they have concerns about how practitioners address the spiritual aspects of care (35). For example, several surveys suggested that over 75% of people identified having a spiritual dimension to their lives (36), and 90% wanted to discuss spirituality and related issues with health and care professionals (37). Patients and carers receiving mental health interventions were concerned with the observable and measureable aspects of care being prioritised over the more subjective aspects of care, such as addressing their spiritual needs (35). Patients were critical of what they considered the 'mechanics of nursing' at the expense of interpersonal and compassionate care.

In contrast to the mental health setting, patients experiencing end of life care believed their spiritual needs were addressed, regardless of religious belief (14). However, patients were often reluctant to raise issues with heath and care professionals whom they perceived as lacking in time to uncover and address issues of a spiritual nature; this resulted in spiritual issues remaining an unmet need for some. Patients at the end of their life had specific spiritual needs as they faced debilitating illness and death. The following insights provide examples of how spiritual care could be enhanced (14):

- Facilitating connections with family, friends and other significant relationships
- Opportunities to feel 'useful' and connected
- Religious experiences such as worship and prayer
- Providing self-help strategies to manage spiritual needs

The Royal College of Physicians End of Life Care Audit: Dying in Hospital (38) highlighted that discussions relating to the spiritual/religious and cultural needs of the dying patient were not often documented. The audit found that it was less likely that spiritual/religious (40%) and cultural needs (28%) would be met in comparison to practical (88%) and psychological needs (71%). The evidence suggests that the needs of dying patients in acute hospital settings are poorly addressed. The recommendations of this audit include the priorities of caring for the dying person and should include an individual plan of care highlighting the spiritual support required.

Research about the experiences of patients of spiritually competent care in other contexts is limited. In the current climate of health and social care where practice is facing intense scrutiny, there is an opportunity to address these issues. Spirituality can be linked to the Dignity in Care and Compassionate Care agendas, which focus on a personalised service, treating the person as an individual. Addressing spirituality, with the understanding that it is integral to a person's sense of identity, a fundamental aspect of human dignity, would support the professional understanding of the patient's unique experiences of their illness and care. Further research is needed about how to do this, but we already know enough to start putting spiritually competent care into practice.

Frameworks for Spiritually Competent Practice and Education

To date there are limited frameworks to support spiritually competent health and care practice. This section explores three frameworks/models for advancing spiritual care in practice drawn from nursing (13), occupational therapy (5) and chaplaincy (39). These frameworks inform our understanding of how spirituality can be operationalized in practice.

The Principle Components Model for Advancing Spirituality

The principle component model for advancing spirituality (13) was developed from a qualitative grounded theory study involving a range of health and care professionals, chaplaincy and the wider public. The

Individuality	The individual experience of spirituality is shaped by 'culture, socialisation, life experience, religious beliefs and institutions' (p.910).
Inclusivity	Refers to adhering to the perceptions and insights of all involved in the delivery of health care and a reflection of the wider community. This component suggests the competencies of the health care professional to address spirituality in their care.
Integrated	Caution against fragmentation, avoiding just another box to tick on the assessment form.
Inter-/intra-disciplinary	This is central to the delivery of spiritual care. Patients advocate 'spirituality is everyone's business' (p.913). Therefore good teamwork is needed.
Innate	Spirituality is innate within individuals, central to a person's being. Words to describe spirituality such as 'sparkle', 'essence', 'inner' and 'makes you, you' have been used (p.914).
Institution	Spirituality is a powerful resource at times of illness and hospitalisation; opportunities to address spiritual needs enhance an individual's sense of well-being. This may be dependent on the setting, for example resources in a hospice take into consideration the achievement of this goal.

Figure 3.1 The Principle Components Model for Advancing Spirituality. (Adapted from McSherry W. *Journal of Clinical Nursing.* 2006; 15:905–917.)

factors inhibiting and advancing spirituality were explored, and the findings supported the development of a model which was grounded in the diverse constraints of practice. Figure 3.1 presents an overview of the model and its components.

The strengths of the model are that it promotes the components of spirituality as central rather than an adjunct to the delivery of care, offering an integrated framework for spiritual care. The model focuses on the patient's experience of spirituality as opposed to the individual practitioner's needs. The involvement of patient's viewpoints in the development of the model addresses many of the criticisms that spirituality in care is developed in isolation from the recipients of care. However, to date the model has not been rigorously evaluated. The model is rich in inter-professional application, however for practitioners needing more profession-specific guidance there are limited frameworks or models available.

Embedding Spirituality: A Framework for Occupational Therapy Practice

The conceptual framework for occupational therapy practice (5) identified the following attributes: development and understanding of one's own spirituality, empathy and positive attitudes towards the belief and values of others, relationship building with patients, person-centred practice valuing the uniqueness of the patients (5,32). The conceptual framework for occupational therapy practice presented in Figure 3.2 shows ways of making links between spirituality, the person and the action of the occupation therapist (5).

The strengths of this framework are that it provides occupational therapists with a tangible structure, developed from the evidence available, to support the practical delivery of good spiritual care. The skills

Occupational therapists' understanding of their own spirituality and positive attitudes, beliefs and values towards spirituality →

Development of an effective therapeutic relationship, sensitive to an individual's beliefs, values and connecting experience →

Unique person-centred engagement in meaningful and purposeful occupations and life situations →

Application of concept analysis findings

Addressing Suffering	Becoming	Meaning	Being	Centeredness	Connectedness	Transcendence
Pain and loss impact on a person's ability to engage in therapeutic intervention	Promoting autonomy, independence and choice through occupations that engage a person in self-healing activities including social and life skills and adaptation to disability	Exploring meaning of personal illness or disruption. Focus on pursuit of goals and interests that enhance quality of life and well-being	Promoting person-centred practice through active listening, valuing beliefs and unique experiences. Allow time to discuss the individuals' values, desires and dreams	Acknowledge an individual's spiritual or religious expressions through meditation, creative visualisation and connection with relationships that create a balance in their life	Connection between the person and the occupational therapist to promote positive well-being outcomes. Facilitating connections with spiritual (and faith) communities (may include prayer and worship)	Existential feelings of a power or force beyond a person. The spiritual aspects of life and care linked to meaning, which may include end of life care, to facilitate positive coping strategies

Person achieves spiritual well-being through engagement with spiritual occupations that address all the spiritual domains →

Figure 3.2 Embedding Spirituality: A Framework for Occupational Therapy Practice. (From Jones J, Topping A, Wattis J, Smith J, *Journal for the Study of Spirituality*. 2016; 6(1):38–57. Copyright British Association for the Study of Spirituality and Maney. Reprinted by permission of Taylor & Francis.)

and attributes required of occupational therapists seeking to practice with spiritual competency have been embedded into the framework. The links between theory and practice support the development of spiritual competency for occupational therapists (6).

The limitation of a profession specific framework or model is the absence of the perspectives of the wider health and care team, and a narrow professional focus influencing patient care. However the strengths are in articulating specific guidance to practitioners supporting their desire for support in operationalizing spirituality and providing a profession specific tool for education. Of course no single professional group has responsibility for spiritual care; rather it should be embedded in all person-centred practice.

Competency Model for the Assessment and Delivery of Spiritual Care

Some chaplains working in palliative care posed the question regarding whose professional responsbility it is to provide spiritual care. A competency framework was developed for all health professionals, offering four developmental levels of involvement in the spiritual care of patients and their carers (39). Figure 3.3 outlines the levels of involvement featured in the competency model for the assessment and delivery of spiritual care.

The framework for involvement has been underpinned by seminars and reflective practice sessions aimed at developing the knowledge, skills and actions at the different levels and enabling staff to be aware of the limits of their competencies. This framework and the accompanying religious and spiritual competencies assessment tools have the potential to provide a transparent process for integrating spirituality into all aspects of care. Whilst this model has been developed for palliative care, it does have transferability to a range of other health and social care settings. The application to the multidisciplinary team supports a deeper understanding of individual members' roles and responsibilities.

A common concern for health and care professionals when discussing how they are prepared for spiritually competent practice is the absence of effective education strategies, or the inclusion of spirituality

Level 1: Staff or volunteers with casual contact with patients, families/carers'	Ensures all staff and volunteers have the basic skills and awareness to refer concerns to the multi-disciplinary team
Level 2: Staff or volunteers requiring contact with patients, families/carers	Enhances level 1 skills, increased awareness of spiritual/religious needs and how to respond Awareness of communication skills needed, personal development and referral of complex cases appropriately
Level 3: Staff or volunteers – members of the multi-disciplinary team	Develops the skills of levels 1 and 2, progressing to the assessment of spiritual/religious need recognizing the complexity of the issues involved
Level 4: Staff or volunteers – primary responsibility for spiritual and religious care	Managing complex needs Required to have a clear personal understanding of their own spirituality/religious beliefs

Figure 3.3 Competency Model for the Assessment and Delivery of Spiritual Care. (Adapted from Gordon T, Mitchell D. *Palliative Medicine*. 2004; 18:646–651.)

in their curriculum (25). Many health and care professionals consider addressing patients' spiritual needs as integral to their practice, however being professionally unprepared leads to feelings of inadequacy and vulnerability (28). Some consider didactic approaches that focus on acquiring academic knowledge to be at variance with the experiential nature of spirituality. The Actioning Spirituality and Spiritual Care Education and Training (ASSET) model (4) provides a problem-based approach to spiritual care education. The focus of the ASSET model is to provide a stand-alone module or as curriculum themes for a course. Embedding experiential learning by developing self-awareness of spiritual understanding and experience were considered essential to developing the spiritual dimensions of nursing. Alternatively, the nursing process has been proposed as a model for teaching spiritual care (40). Effective 'role modelling' in practice has also been proposed as a way for students and junior staff to develop their spiritual competence (41). The effectiveness of role modelling has been demonstrated to impart good clinical competence as skilled health and social care professionals demonstrate compassionate integrity with patients (42). One study involving occupational therapy students suggested that development of the skills required to embed spirituality in practice was enhanced by the enthusiasm and commitment of the academic tutors (43). Occupational therapists may, by the nature of their work, be in a privileged position to provide opportunities to demonstrate spiritual care in practice (6).

Developing Spiritual Competency in Practice

This chapter has highlighted a range of issues relating to spiritual competency across health and care practice. Drawing on the literature and frameworks reviewed, embedding spirituality into health and care practice involves:

- Developing a personal understanding of spirituality
- Acceptance of the individual as unique
- Ability to relate to patients and develop therapeutic relationships
- Cultural competency
- Education
- Reflective practice

Developing a Personal Understanding of Spirituality

It is essential that health and care professionals understand their own spirituality to effectively deliver spiritually competent practice. Valuable skills such as empathy may be associated with a personal appreciation of spirituality. Additionally, a professional's own spirituality can be a resource, providing resilience as a means of coping with the challenges of practice, in particular when caring for the very ill patient (6,44).

Acceptance of the Individual as Unique

Non-judgemental and tolerant acceptance acknowledging the uniqueness of the individual is an essential feature of spirituality and spiritually competent practice (6,45).

Ability to Relate to Patients and Develop Therapeutic Relationships

The development of interpersonal skills to support developing therapeutic relationships with a diverse population of patients is seen as essential to spiritual competency (5). An appreciation of the power differentials between the patient and the practitioner is essential when embedding spirituality into practice. Acknowledging the private and professional interaction is an important skill in maintaining appropriate boundaries. Understanding the vulnerability of the patient is vital when embedding spirituality into care (46). Linked to acknowledging the power differentials and developing effective patient–professional relationships is the ability to understand one's own limitations, and refer on to the most appropriate professional.

Cultural Competency

Cultural competency is integral to delivering spiritually competent care and has been explored in depth earlier in this chapter. Developing a cultural awareness and competency to address the uniquely individual aspects of the patient's experience is essential. Cultural and spiritual competencies are inextricably linked.

Education

The preparation of health and care professionals to practice with spiritual competency is debated (43,47,48). An educational approach which values the experiential nature of spirituality and exposure in practice is favoured. The need for individuals to explore their own understanding of spirituality is challenging in an academic curriculum but can be seen as part of developing reflective practice. Role-modelling in practical work may provide additional opportunities to relate theory to practice. However, using modelling as the only strategy for education relating to spiritual competency places the responsibility on the mentors and placement educators to provide the necessary practice experiences. International studies (47) illuminate the factors contributing to student nurses' development of spiritual care competency. In support of previous studies, an individual's own spirituality (including beliefs and values) is a strong predictor of ability to provide spiritually competent care. The challenge is how to broaden the perspective of students holding a narrow view.

Reflective Practice

Reflection is a requirement of registration for all health and care professionals ensuring practice is critically evaluated and appraised as an essential element of continuing professional development. Reflection increases awareness, enhances professional development and increases confidence and awareness of patients' spiritual needs. Reflective practice provides an excellent opportunity to record confidentially the development of spiritual competency, utilising case studies as examples of spiritually competent care.

Conclusion

Spirituality may appear to be a nebulous topic, shrouded in mystery and contention. In contrast, spiritually competent practice is easier to understand; it is practice which engages the whole person, physical, emotional, mental and spiritual. Spiritually competent practice aims to develop and support the person's sense of meaning and purpose, perhaps through connecting or reconnecting with a community where they experience a sense of well-being. Addressing suffering and supporting the development of coping strategies to improve quality of life congruent with the person's culture, beliefs and values whether religious or not is an important element of spiritually competent practice. Narratives from recent research have been used to illuminate the presence of the constructs contained in spiritually competent practice. Theories and frameworks supporting spiritually competent practice have been presented to guide the reader in developing spiritually competent care and practice that is relevant for their context. Finally, the role of education in preparing spiritually competent health and care practitioners has been briefly considered and is addressed in more depth in Chapter 5. This chapter has presented the case for spiritually competent practice in the context of contemporary health and social care practice by using examples from occupational therapy practice.

References

1. International Council of Nurses. 2012. The ICN Code of Ethics for Nurses. Available at: http://www.icn.ch/who-we-are/code-of-ethics-for-nurses/(accessed 5/2/17).
2. College of Occupational Therapists (COT). *Code of Ethics and Professional Conduct*. London: College of Occupational Therapists; 2015.
3. Health and Care Professions Council (HCPC). Standards of proficiency – Occupational therapists. London: Health and Care Professions Council; 2015.
4. Ellis HK, Narayanasamy A. An investigation into the role of spirituality in nursing. *British Journal of Nursing*. 2009; 18(14):886–890.
5. Jones J, Topping A, Wattis J, Smith J. A concept analysis of spirituality in occupational therapy practice. *Journal for the Study of Spirituality*. 2016; 6(1):38–57.
6. Jones JE. A qualitative study exploring how occupational therapists embed spirituality into their practice. 2016. Unpublished thesis; University of Huddersfield.
7. Van Leeuwen R, Tiesinga LJ, Middel B, Post D, Jochemsen H. The validity and reliability of an instrument to assess nursing competencies in spiritual care. *Journal of Clinical Nursing*. 2009; 18(20):2857–2869.
8. Hodge DR, Baughman LM, Cummings JA. Moving toward spiritual competency: Deconstructing religious stereotypes and spiritual prejudices in social work literature. *Journal of Social Service Research*. 2006; 32(4):211–231.
9. HealthCare Chaplaincy Network. 2016. What is spiritual care and how do we measure it? Available at: http://www.healthcarechaplaincy.org/docs/research/quality_indicators_document_2_17_16.pdf (accessed 5/2/17).
10. Francis R. *Report of the Mid Staffordshire NHS Foundation Trust Public Inquiry*. London: The Stationary Office; 2013.

11. Keogh E. *Review into the Quality of Care and Treatment Provided by 14 Hospital Trusts in England: Overview Report.* NHS England; 2013.

12. Weathers E, McCarthy G, Coffey A. Concept analysis of spirituality: an evolutionary approach. *Nursing Forum.* 2015; 51(2):79–96.

13. McSherry W. The principle components model: a model for advancing spirituality and spiritual care within nursing and health practice. *Journal of Clinical Nursing.* 2006; 15:905–917.

14. Murray SA, Kendall M, Boyd K, Worth A, Benton TF. Exploring the spiritual needs of people dying of lung cancer or heart failure: a prospective qualitative interview study of patients and their carers. *Palliative Medicine.* 2004; 18(1):39–45.

15. Koenig H, King D, Carson VB. *Handbook of Religion and Health.* Oxford, Oxford University Press; 2012.

16. Nagai C. Clinicians' self-assessment of cultural and spiritual competency: working with Asians and Asian Americans. *Community Mental Health Journal.* 2008; 44(4):303–309.

17. Association of Hospice and Palliative Care Chaplains. *Guidelines for Hospice and Palliative Care Chaplaincy* (3rd edition). Association of Hospice and Palliative Care Chaplains; 2013.

18. Clarke J. *Spiritual Care in Everyday Nursing Practice. A New Approach*, Basingstoke: Palgrave Macmillan; 2013.

19. Stewart M. Cultural competence in undergraduate health care education. Review of Issues. *Physiotherapy.* 2002; 88(10):620–629.

20. Hodge DR, Bushfield S. Developing spiritual competence in practice. *Journal of Ethnic and Cultural Diversity in Social Work.* 2007; 15(3–4):101–127.

21. Sessana L, Finnell DS, Underhill M, Chang YP, Peng HL. Measures assessing spirituality as more than religiosity: a methodological review of nursing and health related literature. *Journal of Advanced Nursing.* 2011; 67(8):1677–1694.

22. Office for National Statistics. Religion in England and Wales 2011. Available at: https://www.ons.gov.uk/people-populationandcommunity/culturalidentity/religion/articles/religioninenglandandwales2011/(accessed 5/2/17).

23. The Guardian. People of no religion outnumber Christians in England and Wales – study. Available at: https://www.theguardian.com/world/2016/may/23/no-religion-outnumber-christians-england-wales-study (accessed 8/12/16).

24. Cockell N, McSherry W. Spiritual care in nursing: an overview of published international research. *Journal of Nursing Management.* 2012; 20(8):958–969.

25. Balboni MJ, Sullivan A, Enzinger AC, Epstein-Peterson ZD, Tseng YD, Mitchell C, Niska J, Zollfrank A, VanderWeele TJ, Balboni TA. Nurse and physician barriers to spiritual care provision at the end of life. *Journal of Pain and Symptom Management.* 2014; 48(3):400–410.

26. Ross L, van Leeuwen R, Baldacchino D, Giske T, McSherry W, Narayanasamy A, Downes C, Jarvis P, Schep-Akkerman A. Student nurses' perceptions of spirituality and competence in delivering spiritual care: a European pilot study. *Nurse Education Today.* 2014 ;34(5):697–702.

27. Tiew LH, Creedy DK, Chan MF. Student nurses' perspectives of spirituality and spiritual care. *Nurse Education Today.* 2013; 33(6):574–579.

28. Bursell J, Mayers CA. Spirituality within dementia care: perceptions of health professionals. *The British Journal of Occupational Therapy.* 2010; 73(4):144–151.

29. McSherry W, Jamieson S. The qualitative findings from an online survey investigating nurses' perceptions of spirituality and spiritual care. *Journal of Clinical Nursing.* 2013; 22(21–22):3170–3182.

30. Boschm AG. The meaning of holism in nursing: historical shifts in holistic nursing ideas. *Public Health Nursing,* 1994; 11(5):324–330.

31. Kang C. A psychospiritual integration frame of reference for occupational therapy. Part 1: Conceptual foundations. *Australian Occupational Therapy Journal.* 2003; 50(2):92–103.

32. Egan M, Swedersky J. Spirituality as experienced by occupational therapists in practice. *American Journal of Occupational Therapy.* 2003; 57(5):525–533.

33. Eriksson K. *The suffering human being.* Peterson C, Zetterlund J (eds). Chicago, IL: Nordic Studies Press, 2006.

34. Martinsen K. *Care and Vulnerability.* Oslo: Akribe; 2006.

35. Greasley P, Chiu LF, Gartland RM. The concept of spiritual care in mental health nursing. *Journal of Advanced Nursing.* 2001; 33(5):629–637.

36. Hay D, Hunt K. *Understanding the Spirituality of People Who Don't Go to Church.* Nottingham, UK: Nottingham University; 2000.

37. Sulmasy D. A biopsychosocial-spiritual model for the care of patients at the end of life. *Gerontologist.* 2002; 42(3):24–33.

38. Royal College of Physicians. End of life care audit: dying in hospital. 2016. Available at: https://www.rcplondon.ac.uk/projects/end-life-care-audit-dying-hospital (accessed 17/4/16).

39. Gordon T, Mitchell D. A competency model for the assessment and delivery of spiritual care. *Palliative Medicine.* 2004; 18(7):646–651.

40. Ross LA. Teaching spiritual care to nurses. *Nurse Education Today.* 1996; 16(1): 38–43.

41. The Kings Fund. 2009. Enabling compassionate care in acute hospital settings. Available at: http://www.kingsfund.org.uk/sites/files/kf/field/field_publication_file/poc-enabling-compassionate-care-hospital-settings-apr09.pdf (accessed 5/2/17).

42. Gilbert P, Procter S. Compassionate mind training for people with high shame and self-criticism: overview and pilot study of a group therapy approach. *Clinical Psychology & Psychotherapy.* 2006; 13(6):353–379.

43. Thompson BE, MacNeil C. A phenomenological study exploring the meaning of a seminar on spirituality for occupational therapy students. *American Journal of Occupational Therapy.* 2006; 60,(5):531–539.

44. Hsiao YC, Chiang HY, Chien LY. An exploration of the status of spiritual health among nursing students in Taiwan. *Nurse Education Today.* 2010; 30(5):386–392.

45. McSherry W, Smith J. Spiritual care. In McSherry W, McSherry R, Watson R (eds). *Care in Nursing: Principles, Values and Skills.* Oxford: Oxford University Press; 2012, pp 117–131.

46. Taylor EJ, Park CG, Pfeiffer JB. Nurse religiosity and spiritual care. *Journal of Advanced Nursing.* 70, 11(2014):2612–2621.

47. Ross L, Giske T, van Leeuwen R, Baldacchino, McSherry W, Narayanasamy, Jarvis, P, Schep-Akkerman A. Factors contributing to student nurses'/midwives perceived competency in spiritual care. *Nurse Education Today* 2016; 36:445–451.

48. Attard J, Baldacchino DR, Camilleri L. Nurses' and midwives' acquisition of competency in spiritual care: a focus on education. *Nurse Education Today.* 2014; 34(12):1460–1466.

49. NHS England. A new strategy and vision for nursing, midwifery and care staff. Available at: https://www.england.nhs.uk/nursingvision/ (accessed 8/12/16).

How Two Practitioners Conceptualise Spiritually Competent Practice

4

Melanie Rogers and Laura Béres

Introduction

How can spiritually competent care be conceptualised in ways that are relevant to practice? In this chapter two practitioners focus on how they have approached this question and include insights from their research as well as professional and personal experiences. Melanie, writing from an advanced nurse practitioner and academic background, has many years' experience in addressing and, more recently, researching these issues according to principles of *availability* and *vulnerability*. Laura, as a social work academic, discusses the relevance of her work and research as a *narrative therapist* over many years and the usefulness of the principle of *hospitality*. The authors believe the approaches they use can be relevant to addressing spirituality in all aspects of health and social care.

As discussed in Chapter 3, spiritually competent practice engages a person as a unique spiritual being, in ways which will provide them with a sense of hope, meaning and purpose, connecting or reconnecting with a community where they experience a sense of well-being, addressing suffering and developing coping strategies to improve their quality of life. This includes the practitioner respecting a person's beliefs and values, whether they are religious in foundation or not, and practising with cultural competency (1,2).

This chapter begins by Laura providing descriptions of how utilising narrative therapy skills can support practitioners to provide spiritually competent practice to those they are working with in a variety of settings. Spirituality is often defined as that which provides people with a sense of meaning and purpose in their lives (3,4). These areas of a person's life are easily integrated in narrative therapy because this therapeutic approach provides a structure to conversations that assists people in uncovering and articulating that which gives them meaning, purpose and hope (5,6). The framework of the re-authoring conversation within narrative therapy is particularly helpful in assisting people in articulating meaning and purpose because it focuses on moving away from only problem-saturated storylines and towards a focus on resilience and preferred storylines, which identify closely with an individual's hopes (5,6).

After a few thoughts regarding 'Hospitality,' a framework of 'Availability and Vulnerability' is presented as another way to conceptualise spiritually competent care. It includes fundamental aspects of care many practitioners will be familiar with and can be related to intelligent kindness (7), compassionate care (8), human-to-human connection and the willingness to be open and transparent in practice. Finally, an illustrative narrative is presented and discussed.

Narrative Practices

In *The Narrative Practitioner* (6) Laura describes the importance of the philosophical and political underpinnings of narrative therapy. The originators of the approach, Michael White and David Epston (9), as well as Martin Payne (10) and Laura, have explained the importance of describing the people who come to social services and health services as 'people' rather than 'clients,' 'patients' or 'service users'. They also make their own voices and opinions clear through writing in the first person. This is an attempt to resist the discourses which set up hierarchies between 'professional experts' and people to whom they 'provide services'. Therefore, this section of the chapter is written in a manner congruent with these sensibilities. I (Laura) write in the first person while discussing my work as a narrative therapist. I also describe my therapeutic work as being 'work with people' rather than 'services provided *to*' someone. This aspect of narrative therapy stresses the importance of taking up a therapeutic position that honours the expertise of the lived knowledge of those people who come and participate in therapeutic conversations with narrative therapists. These conversations are as collaborative as possible, keeping in mind the importance of not imposing the therapist's knowledge or values. Narrative therapists may become experts in the process of structuring therapeutic conversations, but the people who come and consult with them are the experts in their own lives and preferences.

Narrative practice is a form of individual, couple and family counselling as well as group and community work (5,9). It is founded on social constructionism, post-modernism and narrative theories which propose that people socially construct a sense of their identity through the stories they tell about themselves to themselves and others. These stories are crafted by stringing together a series of events that have occurred in their lives over time according to a plot or theme, which then have powerful impacts on their beliefs about themselves and how to behave in the world. White points out that there are many more events in any one person's life than ever become narrated into a story (5). He suggests that most events in our lives go by without noting their significance and so lose their power to influence us. When people begin to receive health or social care they have usually come to a point in their lives when they have started to focus on all the events that can be strung together into a problem storyline. They often also think of themselves as a having a problem, or being a problem in one way or another. Much of my clinical practice prior to beginning an academic career involved individual and group counselling with adult survivors of childhood sexual abuse. Most of the people who came to counselling were women, and they would begin by telling me they were 'victims' of sexual abuse. When they felt safe they would recount the events of victimization and those events would create the narrative of their history of childhood sexual abuse. Many of the women would also describe the ongoing effects of their childhood sexual abuse, how they had also been victims of violence whilst dating and had experienced ongoing problematic and sometimes abusive relationships. I particularly remember Lydia telling me she felt like she must have 'V' for 'victim' stamped on her forehead because she felt so much like a 'victim' and so aware that others seemed also to know they could treat her as such.

Narrative approaches have allowed me to work with people in such a way as to move away from 'totalising' accounts which limit their identities according to only problem storylines (6,9,11). By using the framework of a re-authoring conversation in particular, I have been able to assist people in realising that although it is important and healing to give voice to the trauma (12) and break the imposed silence which is often a control tactic of the person who has used abuse, it is also possible to consider all the events in their lives which have fallen outside of the storyline of abuse; there are many events in the lives of 'victims' that have nothing to with victimisation, since there are times where they have avoided or survived abuse and developed resilience. It is possible through the types of questions we ask to show curiosity about the storyline of 'survivor-hood' as well. It is possible to assist people like Lydia to move from feeling trapped by storylines of victim-hood (made up of the series of events linked across time according to the plot of abuse) where their identity is shaped into that of a 'victim', to storylines of 'survivor-hood' where their identity and resulting feelings and thoughts are more like 'survivor'. Lydia, for instance, began to tell me about, and reflect upon, the ways in which she had honed her skills of noticing when the abuse might be imminent and so finding ways to avoid the person who abused her, how she found ways to develop resilience despite the abuse and how she nurtured networks of caring friends even when her non-offending parent did not believe her when her offending parent was charged with sexual abuse; those events began to help her shift towards a focus on her storyline of 'survivor-hood'. During this movement from problem storylines to preferred storylines practitioners ask people they are working with to reflect upon what their emotional and behavioural reactions to events in those storylines might imply about their hopes, dreams and preferences, thereby opening up a focus on spirituality within the therapeutic conversation.

Women I have worked with have found this approach empowering and liberating and have then often moved on to suggest that they would rather their storyline not have anything to do with the abuse at all, not even moving from a storyline of 'victim of abuse' to one of 'survivor of abuse'. It is then possible to assist people in examining their past and present experiences and events and realising there are even more previously un-storied events in their lives which could be narrated according to other plots or themes: the storyline of the development of their careers (one woman focused beautifully on her skills and success as a professional occupational therapist), the storyline of the development of being a good friend, partner and/or mother, or the storyline of sense of self as a new immigrant with a new life in a new country. Lydia used her newfound confidence and sense of herself as not having been deserving of the abuse to apply for victims' compensation through the court system in Canada. When she won a generous settlement she chose to move a significant distance to relocate, buy a small home and develop a whole new storyline where she planned to make new friends, enjoy nature and develop her creativity. These things she had realised over the course of therapy were meaningful to her and had been beginning to develop in importance over the course of many years. These aspects of her life were all related to her spirituality.

Postmodernism has influenced the idea that there are multiple possible storylines in every person's life, rather than focusing on searching for one fundamental 'truth' or 'cause'. Each of the storylines is true, based on events that have occurred, but their weight and significance are further entrenched by the time and attention given them.

Bruner (13) also influenced the development of White and Epston's Narrative Therapy (9) and so the re-authoring conversation is not only made up of a series of events linked over time according to a plot or theme, but also is made up of a landscape of action and a landscape of identity (or landscape of consciousness, as Bruner labelled it). The landscape of action is made up of the 'who', 'what', 'where' and 'when' of the story and the landscape of identity is made up of the 'why' questions which highlight people's hopes, dreams, intentions, purposes and meaning. Asking people why they think they may have responded as they did to a certain event often helps them begin to identify and articulate those things that they hold most precious in their lives which give them meaning and direction: this leads directly to the area of spirituality. (Given the space restrictions in this chapter please see Béres [6] for more about this and further examples.)

All of the narrative practice conversational maps in fact (see 5,6) have a category which assists people in reflecting upon what they think about the effects of certain aspects of their lives, how they judge those effects and why they judge them that way. Although White (5) admits that much of the psychotherapy world warns against asking the 'why' question, because of worries about it sounding judgemental and making people 'defensive,' he has suggested, and I agree, that the 'why' question is perhaps the most important question we can ask because it is what allows us to help people focus on what gives them meaning, purpose and hope: their spirituality. Perhaps counselling approaches have inadvertently moved away from incorporating spirituality as they have taken up the stance which limits the use of 'why'.

This does not mean practitioners should ask questions like, 'Why did you do that?' in a harsh tone, but rather develop gentle ways of asking questions like, 'When you look back at that do you have a sense of what might have motivated you to do that?' 'What were you hoping might be the consequence?' 'Why were you hoping for that consequence, do you think?' 'What does that suggest might be really important and meaningful to you?' These are the types of questions that assist people in uncovering their deeply held beliefs, hopes and dreams. Rather than needing to 'problem solve', White (5) has suggested this can lead to 'problem dissolving' because as people become reminded of, and able to identify, their meaning-making practices and hopes (their spirituality) they are better able to see ways out of problematic situations. These tend to be more in line with their personal beliefs and dreams rather than mutually developed or expert-suggested rational solutions, which may or may not then be followed through.

Hospitality

Hospitality is an important concept for health and social care practitioners, including narrative therapists (6,14,15), and there has been growing interest in it as an ethical manner of engagement in contemporary society (16–20). The tradition of hospitality can be traced back to ancient civilisations and is found in Judaism, Buddhism, Christianity, Islam, Sikhism and other religions. Laura's background and education is in Christian spirituality, so this section is heavily influenced by a particular sixth century Christian monk who wrote about hospitality in a monastic setting. This should not be understood to mean that other traditions do not also have a rich history of contemplating hospitality, nor that professional practitioners need to be affiliated with any religious tradition in order to be able to improve their practice with hospitality. Much in the same way that Buddhist mindfulness has been incorporated into secular professional contexts, so too can hospitality be integrated into a variety of settings.

The Rule of Saint Benedict is helpful for what it offers regarding the concept of hospitality, and, although written in the sixth century, is relevant to health and social care practitioners today. Developing skills of hospitality and the creation of welcoming spaces are skills that can be usefully developed by any practitioner and provide an additional route into spiritually competent practice.

Much of the discussion about Benedict's descriptions of hospitality focuses on the need to be hospitable to the stranger, because in doing so we welcome Christ (14,21, 22). However, Swan (23) and de Waal (22) also describe the need to hold two commitments in tension at the same time. Benedict encourages the provision of a generous reception to guests, but also suggests withdrawing and stepping back in order to ensure the needs of the monastic community are also being met. This ensures that the way of life of the community (silence and prayer) is respected and maintained since it is something about the style of the community that attracts both the members of the community and the guests. 'Benedict is establishing boundaries [. . .] and as any good psychologist would tell us, this is one of the most essential lessons practitioners need to learn' (24, p.156). Directions to hold these two needs in tension may partly be a result of Benedict's focus on developing and maintaining a balanced life, which is also of great importance to health and social care practitioners in order to maintain emotional and physical health, and as a protection against 'burn-out' (15).

Benedict lived in a time of chaos as the Roman Empire was falling, and so his context shares similarities with the chaos many people are experiencing at present. In today's context and with the growing numbers of refugees looking for safety, many people become fearful of strangers and even more fearful of welcoming them into their communities. Practitioners can also sometimes become fearful of people with whom they work, since these people can present in a wide range of manners, from despairing and suicidal to angry and hostile. Homan and Collins-Pratt write, 'When we speak of the depth of hospitality, we are proposing something scary and radical. But it's worth the risk. Unless we find and practice ways of hospitality we will grow increasingly hostile' (18, p.xxii). They use the image of preparing a table as an overall metaphor for a type of hospitality that '... seeps into your soul and shapes your identity. We can give this kind of hospitality to each other only if we take the time to prepare sheltering places around us' (18, p.114). They say,

> The table, for the teacher or social worker, is her or his desk. Whatever the specific physical structures of your work might be, you give something to others from them. You create a space for others because work is always for the service of others (18, p.115).

Contemporary health and social care practitioners create space to work with others and may develop further skills in spiritually competent practice through reflecting on Benedict's instructions about how to bow to welcome guests, read, pray and eat with them, provide adequate space for quiet and bedding for comfortable sleep. Health and social care practitioners should not necessarily be praying with people who come to consult them, but this list reminds practitioners of the need to attend holistically to the people they see, responding to emotional, physical, social, intellectual and spiritual aspects of their lives (23).

Availability and Vulnerability are two other concepts, derived from a contemporary dispersed Christian community (a monastic community where members live separately), which also offer much for integrating spiritually into competent practice.

Availability and Vulnerability

Spiritually competent practice is innately human and influenced by context and emotional engagement. It can be operationalised through a framework of availability and vulnerability (25). Spiritually competent practice fundamentally focuses on relationship and connection with those we are working with and demands a level of emotional involvement within professional boundaries.

The development of this framework for operationalising spiritually competent practice arose from an enquiry into the spiritual dimensions of primary care advanced nurse practitioners' (ANPs') consultations (25). This phenomenological study took the form of two in-depth interviews 18 months apart with eight experienced ANPs. During the first interview participants were asked to talk about their clinical practice, how they defined and operationalised spirituality in addition to exploring how they defined availability and vulnerability and whether this related to spirituality for them. The second interview explored spiritual dimensions of their practice in more detail and brought in a concept of 'Availability and Vulnerability' derived from the Northumbria Community's Rule of Life to see how this related to their own view of spirituality. The Northumbria Community (NC) is a dispersed Christian monastic community which Melanie encountered 20 years ago. The NC follow a Rule of Life of 'Availability and Vulnerability', like a modern-day simplified version of the rule of Benedict discussed above. All the participants viewed availability and vulnerability as integral to their practice, and over 18 months of engagement the majority of participants went on to see availability and vulnerability as a useful way of operationalising spirituality (25). They were able to see availability and vulnerability broadly outside of a religious framework in much the same way as secular versions of Buddhist mindfulness have been widely applied in health care practice.

Rogers' Availability and Vulnerability Framework for Spiritually Competent Care

This framework is intended to support spiritually competent practice. It has been broken down into aspects of availability (Box 4.1) and vulnerability (Box 4.2) to aid understanding and application to practice.

1. **Availability to ourselves**

To be available to ourselves continuing as practitioners to be self-reflective and self-accepting, embracing spirituality (broadly defined as understanding of one's meaning, purpose and direction in life) as key to our inner journey (15,25).

Part of this aspect of availability is the recognition that much of our work with others has an emotional impact. At times this can be extensive and on some occasions it can lead to burn-out (26). Taking time to

Box 4.1 Availability

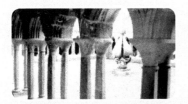
To be available to ourselves; continuing as a practitioner to be self-reflective and self-accepting, embracing spirituality (broadly defined as understanding of one's meaning, purpose and direction in life) as key to our inner journey.

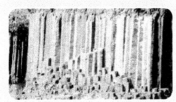
To be welcoming to those in our care, offering time, acceptance and understanding whilst being truly present and listening attentively.

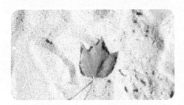
To offer care and concern for those in our care through active participation, creating a safe place to tell their story as it is.

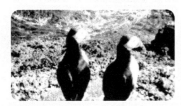
To be available to develop professional practice in response to the needs of the community and those in our care.

reflect on the way we choose to practice and how our values and beliefs affect our practice allows us to consider whether they are expressed congruently, and if not, how we can address this. It ensures we have time to consider whether we are giving too much to others whilst not recognising our own needs. It gives us time to nurture our inner selves and adapt our practice, if needed. It also allows us recognise when we are giving too much of ourselves and risking 'burn-out'. This is a risk for practitioners who often put their heart into caring. Wright suggests it is unusual for burn-out to occur out of the blue and for many it is a gradual process over years (27). There are external factors influencing burn-out such as excessive pressure of work, poor support and leadership (28). Being fully aware of the boundaries within practice, continuing to reflect on practice and being self-aware are protective (see Chapter 6 for further discussion). Experienced practitioners, whilst remaining within their professional codes of conduct, sometimes recognise the need for boundaries to be flexible in order to be able to work effectively.

Self-reflection, self-acceptance, self-care and supervision are vital for healthy relationships in the helping professions. Self-acceptance is important before we can truly accept others as they are (29). Being comfortable with self and being at home in one's skin are foundational for authentic work with patients. Vanier (29, p.23) states that 'People reach maturity as they find the freedom to be themselves, and to claim, accept and love their own personal story, with all its brokenness and beauty'. By consistently reflecting on our journey the authentic self becomes an agent for increased compassion and honest relationships through true self-acceptance.

2. Availability to Others through Welcome

Being welcoming to those in our care; offering time, acceptance and understanding whilst being truly present and listening attentively' (15,25).

This is strongly related to the theme of hospitality discussed above. How we begin a relationship influences how it develops. Taking time to introduce ourselves, explain how long we have together and provide a safe, open environment where we are fully present and listen attentively are all important. By consciously welcoming people who come to see us and by being open and willing to be available to them and to truly listen, the ground is laid for a mutual exchange based on equality and acceptance. A key component of this is truly listening. Nouwen (30) linked this to acceptance. He suggested that true listening was not just letting someone speak but paying full attention to what they were saying, what they were not saying and who they were. Expanding upon this, he wrote 'the beauty of listening is that those who are listened to start feeling accepted, start taking their words more seriously and discovering their true selves. Listening is a form of spiritual hospitality ...' (30, p.85).

3. Availability to Others through Caring

To offer care and concern for those in our care through active participation, creating a safe place to tell their story as it is (15,25).

To truly offer care and concern, the ability to 'hold' another without becoming overwhelmed or enmeshed is important. As practitioners mature in their work they recognise that some approaches to care taught in training can be rigid and limiting. One of the most powerful interactions is just 'being' with another and offering care and compassion. Martisen (31) and Erikkson (32) suggest that caring for others is a form of 'neighbourly love' denoted by the Latin word *'caritas'* This is also consistent with the humanistic term *unconditional positive regard* which denotes acceptance and support of a person regardless of what the person says or does (see Chapter 1). This deep care and concern for another necessitates the practitioner working in a way that is moral, practical and professional (33).

4. Availability to Develop Practice

To be available to develop practice in response to the needs of the community and those in our care (15,25).

In order to develop practice there needs to be an awareness of the needs of those in our care and also in the communities where we practice. This enables our work to be dynamic and responsive whilst recognising the limits of health and social care in the current financial climate. Many practitioners, once qualified, go on to undertake specialist training. One example is the integration of narrative therapy skills into practice. Having the ability to be responsive in our work is professionally satisfying and should always focus on the needs of those in our care.

Availability Summary

Throughout my own practice and research, I (Melanie) have found that availability is a powerful mediator for spiritually competent practice. The synergistic relationship that exists between the practitioner and those in their care is a powerful vehicle for building authentic relationships. Practitioners need to be willing to constantly reflect on their own practice, the emotional impact their work has on them and whether they are able to offer the care and concern necessary to those with whom they work. Being intentionally available involves making a choice to offer a safe place, to be able to listen and be fully present, listening attentively to help those in our care feel accepted and valued as they are.

Aspects of availability will be easily understandable for many practitioners and are part of good professional practice. The concept of vulnerability embraces the humanistic concept of genuineness, congruence or authenticity (see Chapter 1). However, it goes beyond this and into potentially controversial areas. Initially vulnerability may be viewed negatively, denoting weakness or being at risk of harm. Within the present framework, vulnerability is seen as being intentional; choosing to be authentic, being willing to be challenged, being teachable and being willing to be an advocate for those in our care. It also includes a degree of humility and willingness to learn from those in our care. Recognising the privilege of being part of people's deepest struggles connects deeply to spirituality and enables a reframing of vulnerability as an intentional openness to the suffering of others.

Box 4.2 Vulnerability

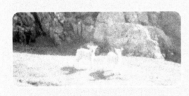

To be teachable; accepting the vulnerability of our role and the reality that within our work we will never 'know all'.

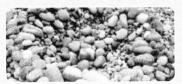

To be willing to embrace accountability, engaging in supervision and reflection. Being willing to admit mistakes and being receptive to constructive criticism. To be willing to share uncertainty with those in our care and act in a way which is open, honest and transparent, working within personal and professional limitations.

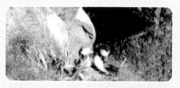

To be willing to be an advocate for those in our care. If necessary questioning authority, being honest and truthful with the best interests of the those in our care at heart.

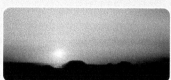

To be vulnerable and authentic in the approach to those in our care.

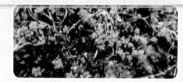

To be willing to be challenged and questioned without defensiveness.

1. Embracing Vulnerability by Being Teachable

To be teachable; accepting the vulnerability of our role and the reality that within our work we will never 'know all' (15,25).

Health and social care practice is constantly evolving. We will never know it all and need to be willing to recognise that, no matter how experienced we become, learning and development remain ongoing needs. The willingness to be open to new knowledge, experiences and skills aids practice. Being able to work within limitations and refer on when necessary is part of what enables those in our care to trust us. One of the advantages to working in multi-professional teams is the sharing of expertise, but this demands a willingness to accept when we need help ourselves.

2. Willingness to Be Accountable to Others

To be willing to embrace accountability, engaging in supervision and reflection. Being willing to admit mistakes and being receptive to constructive criticism. To be willing to share uncertainty with those in our care and act in a way which is open, honest and transparent, working within personal and professional limitations (15,25).

Being able to recognise when we are out of our depth, not helping someone or in need of support for ourselves is healthy. It denotes an understanding of the complexities of our work which is multi-faceted and enables us to be authentic and open. Accountability is fundamental to practice. Both colleagues and those in our care need to be able to trust us. I have found that the patients I work with value my honesty when I say I am unable to offer a diagnosis and need to refer on to someone else. I may say something like 'I'm not sure what is going on here but let's try this and see how things go', 'I'm going to ask a colleague to see you as I don't have much experience of ...', or 'What do you think is going on here?' This enables accountability to those in our care and openness often fosters trust. Part of my authentic practice is also being willing to recognise if I have made a mistake. It is important that we never feel we 'know it all' and that we recognise the need for further training, education and the support of colleagues. Miller (34) quotes Thomas Merton, who reminds us that 'the only mistake is one you don't learn from'.

3. Being Willing to Be Vulnerable by Advocating for Patients

Being willing to be an advocate for those in our care. If necessary, questioning authority, being honest and truthful with the best interests of those in our care at heart (15,25).

Advocacy is a common aspect of our practice. Being willing to speak up for those who feel they don't have a voice, or those who are unable to advocate for themselves can be a challenge. Having the integrity to gently confront colleagues or the organisational structures and guidelines that sometimes inhibit care can result in the practitioner feeling very vulnerable. Those we advocate for often recognise that we value and really listen to them when we stand up for them and 'put our heads above the parapet'.

4. Vulnerability and Authenticity

To be vulnerable and authentic in the approach to those in our care (15,25).

In order to connect with another fully, authenticity is necessary. The goal with this aspect of vulnerability is to put building of the professional relationship with the patient above concerns for one's own reputation. Professional reputation is important, of course, but the goal is not to put value in being a professional above the human-to-human connection with the patient. Relationships based upon care for patients are fundamental to holistic practice. This concept parallels the work of Ballatt and Campling (7), who focus on intelligent kindness as a dynamic that should be at the heart of care which humanises health care (see Chapter 9). Like Martinson (31), they recognise concepts similar to caritas and identify the roots of kindness in 'kinship', our shared humanity. Within their descriptions of intelligent kindness there is recognition of the need to connect to others in human-to-human interactions. This can seem risky, as to do this, practitioners need to be vulnerable and authentic, which can lead to being hurt or misunderstood.

5. Vulnerability and Openness to Challenge

To be willing to be challenged and questioned without defensiveness (15,25).

Being willing to be challenged and questioned about our practice is positive. Being able to accept constructive criticism enables practitioners to develop personally and professionally. This aspect of vulnerability necessitates maturity and resilience to be able to see criticism as developmental rather than destructive. Of course, this partly depends on how the criticism is delivered. Within this aspect of vulnerability, humility about our professional standing or reputation is important. This does not mean we negate our professional standing but that we focus on the relationship with those in our care which is often the most fundamental aspect of our work.

Vulnerability Summary

Some of the aspects of vulnerability described above are expected aspects of our work and may not be considered exclusively as characteristics of spiritually competent practice. However, vulnerability expressed in our willingness to be authentic and acknowledging the need to connect as human to human with all our insecurities, frailties, mistakes and limitations, can radically change our work. Whilst maintaining our professionalism, we can learn to be open about our limitations. People we work with and care for will generally respect this. Recognising our need to continue learning and developing and being accountable for our practice helps us acknowledge we, like our patients, are fallible and human and moves the relationship to a more equal footing.

Utilising availability and vulnerability as a framework for spiritually competent practice can have a major impact on practitioners and those we care for. Availability and vulnerability support practice in a way which is freeing and adaptable, recognising the patients' and our own spirituality. Many of the aspects described are simply elements of good professional practice yet when brought together they connect deeply to spiritually competent practice. There is recognition of the other as fully human and connected to us through humanity. Inherent worth is seen and acknowledged in those we care for and signified by a willingness to be present ('being') and attentive rather than focusing on 'doing'. Spiritually competent practice can also be evident in the tasks we carry out, as these can be offered in a way which values the other, is compassionate and kind. Being together, being authentic, being vulnerable enough to accept our limitations and mistakes is fundamental to spiritually competent practice.

The following narrative (Box 4.3) connects deeply with spiritually competent practice. It is a beautiful and powerful example of spirituality in practice revealing how availability and vulnerability enabled a human connection to develop which profoundly affected both practitioner and patient. All names and identifying data and the details have been changed to ensure confidentiality and anonymity. Consent has been obtained to use the verbatim quotes of the ANP who was part of a recently completed study (25).

Box 4.3 Illustrative Narrative

Abi was a 15-year-old girl when she began to see Ana, an ANP, after being diagnosed with a mental health problem. Abi was the same age as Ana's own daughter, which immediately caused her to consider how she would feel if this was her own daughter:

> I had to be kind of aware of that and keep that at a distance, you know because you respond as a clinician but you also respond as a mother.

For Ana this brought about a connection based on empathy and care which developed over the next few years and became more emotionally complex when Abi's mum died suddenly. It was clear that Ana felt deeply as she said:

> I feel myself getting emotional about it as I talk, so excuse me, but she's only 16 and her mum died. She is the same age as my daughter you see and that was really difficult … I just thought this is too terrible for words. I know people die all the time but it was just too

close you know and then I thought 'how am I going to see her again, I am going to fall apart completely'. I was worried about how I would react and of course how she would feel and how I would deal with all of that and I remember the woman who I see for supervision she said 'well can you carry on seeing her?' and I said 'well how can I not?' You know I couldn't not see her obviously even if it was difficult for me to see her so I did and it was difficult.

Ana acknowledged clearly her care for Abi and her shock and sadness that she had lost her mum. She also acknowledged that she felt a level of responsibility for her which she reflected on after Abi eventually went on to a university overseas and received support from there:

I actually feel quite relieved that she is getting that support there now because while ever she wasn't doing that although I knew she was no longer my responsibility in that sense, you can't just let that go can you and I still see her in the holidays and e-mail her occasionally but there feels like there is a slight distance coming there now which I feel is actually quite appropriate.

Although a clear human connection was present which involved deep care, empathy and compassion it was rarely verbally acknowledged until towards the end of their consultations together as Ana felt strongly that she needed to maintain her professional boundaries, although she acknowledged how much Abi meant to her:

I had to be very, very careful in this to – I don't know how you can explain it – to have a level of openness and involvement but without her having known I guess how personal it was or without us ever acknowledging that in a way because I think she knew that I had children her age. She never mentioned it and obviously I never mentioned it until the very last time I saw her when she went to America and she asked me about my children which was interesting really and I could talk about it then briefly but it wouldn't have been appropriate to have talked about it at any other time but there was that awareness that she was interested in my life. It's how you can be of help and value to a person in that position and I think when I was thinking about this … you have got to be very careful that the consultation doesn't in any way become about you. That would be the risk wouldn't it that in being open and I am talking more generally here than just with Abi in being open you mustn't ever cross that line where it becomes too much about me and not about them anymore.

Ana and Abi navigated not just living with and addressing a mental health problem with all its complexities but also the significant loss of Abi's mum. They continued to have a healthy practitioner and patient relationship where there was a deep connection but where Ana ensured a professional boundary was in place despite many conflicting emotions around the desire to mother this girl. Connection gave Abi a sense of stability and consistency for a number of years before she went to University, and it is clear that this meant a lot to her as she still contacts Ana occasionally when she comes home for holidays. Her relationship with Ana appears to have been hugely significant.

Abi often reflected to Ana her existential angst and search for hope, meaning and purpose in her life, especially after losing her mum. Her need to explore this was the focus of many of their consultations and she eventually made the decision to go to University to study. Her journey with a mental health problem and loss at such an early age provoked many of the questions about life and revealed a spiritual need to Ana for which she was able to allow space for exploration in their therapeutic interactions.

Application and Discussion of the Framework to the Vignette Including Related Concepts

Availability (Including Hospitality)

Abi's story (Box 4.3) illustrates the integration of spiritually competent care in Ana's practice. When interviewed, Ana spoke about her belief that spirituality was innate and part of being human. In her relationship with Abi she could not be anything but 'human', whilst recognising the boundaries of practice so the consultations remained about Abi and not Ana. Ana was able to be self-reflective throughout her relationship with Abi and acknowledged the deep emotional repercussions that occurred because she chose to be available and vulnerable with Abi.

Ana made a choice to offer Abi a welcoming, safe place where she could be truly herself and share her struggles and also the loss of her mother. She built a relationship with Ana based on trust and respect. Ana worked with Abi to be deeply present throughout her struggles, showing care and concern.

There were many occasions when Abi lost hope, meaning and purpose and Ana was also challenged personally in these areas. Yet even though Ana was offered the opportunity to stop seeing Abi she continued to hold hope for her and chose to continue seeing her until she left for University.

The consultations with Abi lasted over several years and had a deep impact on Ana which at times was difficult to manage. Through supervision and taking care of her own needs she was able to traverse these difficulties and maintain an approach to care based on human connection, and deep care and compassion.

Ana was incredibly self-reflective and self-accepting during her relationship with Abi. She recognised the importance of spiritually competent practice but in order for her to continue to be available she needed to reflect with her supervisor about her own needs and the impact the relationship had on her. She recognised what was important in her own life and, in her work with Abi, she tried to support her to find meaning and purpose, especially when her life felt hopeless.

Ana offered Abi a safe place to be able to talk openly about her fears, anxieties and daily struggles with a mental health problem and then the loss of her mum. Ana was able to be fully present in her interactions with Abi despite the difficult emotions she experienced and her deep empathy for Abi. Over several years Abi felt accepted and understood.

The safe place that Ana created for Abi was based on recognising how alone Abi felt and the inner turmoil and distress she experienced. Ana offered care and concern for Abi throughout her interactions. She was able to welcome Abi's story as it was without feeling the need to adapt it to make it easier to deal with.

In response to her work with Abi, Ana decided that to develop her practice she would pursue further training in working with mental health problems. She recognised the increasing incidence of mental health problems in primary care and used her training to develop a new service for patients.

Vulnerability

Ana recognised her need to learn in her work with Abi. She often worked with significant physical, emotional and social complexities in her clinical practice. She often engaged in more study to increase her knowledge base, but key to her practice was the ability to ask for guidance from her supervisor who was able to offer insights, guidance and support. Throughout this process she was able to be vulnerable with her supervisor knowing she held Ana's best interest as paramount. Ana engaged in supervision to be able reflect on her practice with Abi and other patients in her care. She found that within supervision she could explore her emotional responses in a safe way which enabled her to continue to work with Abi.

Ana on several occasions needed to be an advocate for Abi. When Abi applied to University Ana needed to write a supporting letter in view of her medical history. There were concerns about offering her place at University, so Ana ensured that an honest report was provided which focused on Abi's resilience and recovery.

Ana's values and beliefs about her clinical work were clearly evident when she described the experience she had caring for Abi. She 'gave' of herself for many years in order for Abi to feel she had a safe place to be herself and share her struggles. Ana showed her care by continuing to see Abi even when she found it emotionally painful herself. Although she did not share how she felt with Abi, she remained authentic in her approach and during supervision explored her own needs.

This final aspect of vulnerability was evident for Ana when her supervisor asked her if she should stop seeing Abi. During supervision they were able to explore Ana's feelings and her conflict between her own needs and those of Abi without defensiveness.

Through this vignette spirituality can be further understood through its relationship to availability and vulnerability. This vignette shows the innateness of spirituality mediated through human-to-human connection. The outcome for Abi was that she regained hope, meaning and purpose and for Ana; holding out hope for Abi and seeing her recovery gave her a sense of meaning and purpose personally and professionally.

Conclusion

We have offered approaches which we have found helpful in providing spiritually competent practice. At the heart of these is the relationship built between practitioners and people we work with. Spirituality is about what gives people hope, meaning and purpose, and spiritually competent practice is about assisting people to become clearer about what it is that gives them hope, meaning and purpose. Human-to-human connection based on hospitality, availability and a willingness to be vulnerable in the therapeutic relationship facilitates this. Specific approaches from narrative therapy can then integrate questions and interactions which will assist the people we work with in moving away from problem-saturated accounts of themselves and developing an account providing them with a new sense of meaning and purpose. We have described specific approaches that can help practitioners to recognise that much of their practice may already be spiritually competent. Narrative therapy is an established approach that is particularly suited to helping people find and articulate their hopes, and what gives them a sense of meaning and purpose in their lives. The principles of availability, vulnerability and hospitality, found in many religious and philosophical traditions, provide a setting for approaching these issues. Spiritually competent practice is not esoteric; it is about developing professional skills and models of practice that reduce unnecessary professional 'distance'. It is about caring about the whole person and taking into account everything that contributes to a person's sense of meaning and quality of life. It is good practice!

References

1. Rogers M, Wattis, J. Spirituality in nursing practice. *Nursing Standard*. 2015; 29(39) 51–57.
2. Jones J, Topping A, Wattis J, Smith J. A concept analysis of spirituality in occupational therapy practice. *Journal for the Study of Spirituality*. 2016; 6(1):38–57.
3. Canda E. Spirituality, diversity, and social work practice. *Social Casework*. 1988; 69(4):238–247.
4. Cook C, Powell A, Sims A (eds). *Spirituality and Psychiatry*. Glasgow: Royal College of Psychiatrists Publications; 2009.
5. White, M. *Maps of Narrative Practice*. New York: Norton; 2007.
6. Béres L. *The Narrative Practitioner*. London: Palgrave-Macmillan; 2014.
7. Ballatt J, Campling P. *Intelligent Kindness – Reforming the Culture of Healthcare*. London: Royal College of Psychiatrists; 2013.
8. Department of Health. Compassion in practice. Nursing, midwifery and care staff. Our vision and strategy. https://www.england.nhs.uk/wp-content/uploads/2012/12/compassion-in-practice.pdf (accessed 1/2/17). London: Department of Health.
9. White M, Epston D. *Narrative Means to Therapeutic Ends*. New York: Norton; 1990.
10. Payne, M. *Narrative Therapy, Second Edition: An Introduction for Counsellors*. London: Sage; 2006.
11. Duvall J, Béres L. *Innovations in Narrative Therapy: Connecting Practice, Training, and Research*. New York: Norton; 2011.
12. Duvall J, Béres L. Movement of identities: a map for therapeutic conversations about trauma. In Brown C, Augusta-Scott T (eds). *Narrative Therapy: Making Meaning, Making Lives* Thousand Oaks, CA: Sage; 2007, pp 229–250.
13. Bruner J. *Actual Minds, Possible Worlds*. Cambridge, MA: Harvard University Press; 1986.
14. Aman J. Therapist as host: making my guests feel welcome. *International Journal of Narrative Therapy and Community Work*. 2006; 3:3–10.
15. Béres L (ed). *Practicing Spirituality: Reflections on Meaning-Making in Personal and Professional Contexts*. London: Palgrave-Macmillan; 2017.
16. Cotter J. *Love Rekindled: Practising Hospitality*. Evesham: Cairns Publications and Sheffield: Arthur James; 1996.
17. Derrida J, Dufourmantelle A. *Of Hospitality: Anne Dufourmantelle Invites Jacques Derrida to Respond*. Lauray RB (trans). Stanford, CA: Stanford University Press; 2000.
18. Homan OSB D, Collins Pratt L. *Radical Hospitality: Benedict's Way of Love*. Glasgow: Wild Goose Publications; 2007.
19. Kramer KT. Radical hospitality. *America*. 2011; 204(6):9.
20. Pearson PM. Hospitality to the stranger: Thomas Merton and St. Benedict's exhortation to welcome the stranger as Christ. *American Benedictine Review*. 2011; 62(1):27–41.
21. Chittester OSB J. *The Rule of Benedict: Insights for the Ages*. New York: Crossroad; 2004.
22. de Waal E. *A Life-giving Way: A Commentary on the Rule of St. Benedict*. Collegeville; MN: The Liturgical Press; 1995.
23. Swan L. *Engaging Benedict: What the Rule can Teach us Today*. Notre Dame, IN: Ave Maria Press; 2005.
24. Swinton J. *Spirituality and Mental Health Care: Rediscovering a 'forgotten' Dimension*. London: Jessica Kingsley; 2001.
25. Rogers M. Spiritual dimensions of advanced nurse practitioner consultations in primary care through the lens of availability and vulnerability. a hermeneutic enquiry. Doctoral thesis, University of Huddersfield; 2016.
26. Cherniss C. *Staff Burnout: Job Stress in the Human Services*. Beverly Hills, CA: Sage; 1980.

27. Wright S. *Reflections on Spirituality and Health*. London: Whurr; 2005.

28. Leineweber C, Westerlund H, Chungkham HS, Lindqvist R, Runesdotter S, et al. Nurses' practice environment and work-family conflict in relation to burn out: a multilevel modelling approach. *PLoS ONE*. 2014; 9(5):e96991.

29. Vanier J. *Drawn into the Mystery of Jesus through the Gospel of John*. Ottawa, Canada: Novalis; 2004.

30. Nouwen H. *Bread for the Journey: Reflections for Every day of the Year*. London: Darton, Longman and Todd; 1996.

31. Martinsen K. *Care and Vulnerability*. Oslo: Akribe; 2006.

32. Lindström U, Nyström L, Zetterlund J. Theory of caritative caring. In Alligood M (ed). *Nursing Theorists and their Work* (8th edition). Maryland Heights, MO: Elsevier; 2014.

33. Alvsvåg H. Philosophy of caring. In Alligood M (ed). *Nursing Theorists and their Work* (8th edition). Maryland Heights, MO: Elsevier; 2014.

34. Miller T. The Northumbria community: who are we? 2014. Available at: http://www.northumbriacommunity .org/who-we-are/ (accessed 4/6/14).

How Can Spirituality Be Integrated in Undergraduate and Postgraduate Education?

5

Michael Snowden and Gulnar Ali

This chapter explores the perceived challenges presented to those educators attempting to incorporate spiritual care within curricula. Although the discussion and solutions presented focus primarily on nursing education, other health and social care professions face similar challenges and consequently the recommendations presented are transferable and applicable to other groups.

Why Should Spirituality Be Part of a Curriculum?

The notion of spiritual care as the promotion and purpose of life as an ideal has been embraced by the nursing profession since the time of Florence Nightingale. Over the past three decades its distinct association with the development of holistic care has ensured that spirituality and its application to the development of care has become a topical issue debated by scholars and practitioners alike.

The Royal College of Nursing (RCN) (1) and the North American Nursing Diagnosis Association (2) (NANDA) place due emphasis upon the importance of spiritual and religious care in promoting health and well-being in the context of holistic care. However, as illustrated by Ali et al (3), assessment and care planning do not always take these factors into account; neither are spiritual aspects of care always made explicit in standards associated with promoting excellence in care.

Approaching Spirituality

Nursing philosophy has, as a central tenet, the concept of holism placing emphasis upon the multi-dimensional nature of the human. Person-centeredness, or individualised care, is nothing new in education;

attention to the spiritual aspects of care has been advocated (4) for over 30 years as a way of ensuring care is truly holistic, with calls to integrate spiritual care within nursing education over a similar period (5–10).

However, there is no consensus about how this can be achieved. The theory and practice of teaching and education (pedagogy) are not well developed in this area and the presence of spirituality in curricula is variable. As a consequence, students often feel ill-prepared for practice in this area.

Spiritual assessment is a recognised part of good nursing care (1,2), yet there are issues in embedding spirituality within the nursing curriculum and teaching practice (9,11). Ali et al (3), following a detailed and comprehensive literature review, asserted that reasons for this were complex, including the dominance of reductionist and positivist views. However, approaches to spirituality are characterised by a completely different set of assumptions. These result in a complex, emergent and developing concept of self which exists only when contextualised in an holistic manner (3). The positivistic focus of existing nursing education (7,8,12) dominates what subjects are taught and how they are taught. The lack of role clarity and expertise among educators, and workload priorities compound the deficiency (13).

Whilst NANDA (2), the RCN (1) and other agencies have recognised the importance of assessing spiritual care needs and this is considered to be an established part of global nursing practice, spiritual care receives little attention in nursing education (9–11). In the United Kingdom (UK), there exists an anomalous relationship between academic and clinical policy documents. The RCN (1) offers a significant resource on spirituality in nursing care for both learners and practitioners but the UK's Nursing and Midwifery Council (14) enforces a statutory code for professional practice without any specific mention of spirituality. The USA and Ireland are cited as having similar conflicts (10,15). In contrast, this is not the case in medicine, where the UK's General Medical Council (16) mandates spiritual factors should be considered as part of the assessment process.

Why Is Spirituality Lacking in the Curriuculum?

Over the last three decades there have been a number of calls (3,7) to integrate spiritual care into nursing education. However, there is no consensus about how this can be achieved and there is a lack of consistent integration within the curriculum. The reasons for this are far from clear. There are conceptual, philosophical, cultural, political, linguistic and epistemological challenges to understanding spirituality and its relationship to practice (5,10,12,17,18). These conceptual challenges present a barrier to successful integration.

Defining spirituality is a complex issue explored elsewhere in this book. Palmer (19) asserts that 'spirituality is an elusive word with a variety of definitions, some compelling, some wifty, some downright dangerous' (p.377). That complexity is a background to educational endeavour. Spirituality is often regarded as synonymous with religion but it is a separate though related concept. Religious expression can be confined to particular belief systems, a formal expression of getting connected with the sacred; institutional and measurable in terms of frequency of attending rituals and offering prayers. Spirituality may be understood as the personal, inner, informal and emotional aspect of connecting with oneself, the environment or with the sacred (20) and influences internal motives and resilience factors including underlying hope. Cooper et al (21) suggest that 'broad existential definitions that deliberately separate any relationship between spirituality and religion or theology, [leave] the concept of spirituality open to be confused with the psycho-social' (p.1058). This vagueness contributes to a perception that spirituality can be covered within other aspects of the curricula, where it can be taught alongside concepts such as personal values, psychological or cultural issues, resulting in it becoming an increasingly diluted and vague aspect of learning. This lack of specificity presents a distinct challenge to educators. With the ever-increasing popularity of modularisation within curricula and scales of economy in higher education, spirituality as a learning concept becomes edged out by other more positivist learning opportunities, with distinct measurable and quantifiable outputs. The prioritisation of positivistic care approaches over humanistic care, a lack of transcultural awareness as well as financial and time constraints, all affect nursing education and practice, diminishing the perceived importance of spirituality within the curriculum. Yilmaz and Gurler (15) assert that greater application is required to integrate spirituality successfully within the curriculum.

There are numerous challenges and issues that impede the identity of spirituality within the curriculum (3,13,17). As well as problems of definition, lack of confidence and expertise in educators, political influences on institutional policies, challenges from multicultural faith systems, professional constraints and work load priorities, personal bias and experience all contribute to confusion and lack of clarity within the curriculum. Studies (9,11,15) exploring learners' views revealed that the existing nursing curriculum does not appear to adequately prepare nurses to connect with patients' existential and spiritual dimensions. This appears to be due to inadequate explanation, insufficient mentorship and deficiency in articulating spirituality and spiritual care needs. Barss (22) identified barriers which included the lack of recognition of the relationship between general health and spiritual care, insufficient time for learners to provide spiritual care due to prioritising physical complaints and role ambiguity of both learners and educators when offering support in cases of spiritual distress.

There is little research available to nurse educators that identifies the competencies that need to be developed to ensure that future practitioners are able to identify and respond to spiritual care needs (24) confidently. At present, there is a lack of incorporation of spiritual competence into nursing standards (14), though research attempts have been made to define the competencies required (see Chapter 1). In addition, with reference to the existing nursing curriculum, Benner et al (7) claimed that current nursing education does not adequately prepare nurses to connect with patients' existential and spiritual dimensions.

McSherry and Draper (17) identified certain barriers to education in this area. They included:

1. The time needed to develop skills for assessing spiritual care needs of patients
2. The need for competent mentoring for learners approaching spiritual care issues
3. Managerial problems related to financial implications
4. The work load on nursing educationists in revising the existing curriculum
5. A lack of acknowledgement of the role of cultural diversity in this area

Although the article referred to barriers with particular reference to the UK 30 years ago, similar issues still need to be addressed (10). Timmins et al (11), as recently as 2014, found that whilst nursing textbooks offered some guidance and direction around spiritual care, few provided relevant detail on spirituality, failing to discuss various definitions or explore the relationship of spirituality to religion.

However, there are examples of good practice that educators can draw upon to develop teaching and learning strategies. Cone and Giske (23) utilised role-modelling and mentoring to support learners in developing insights in this area. More formal models have been developed by Barss (22) introducing the TRUST model (Traditions, Reconciliation, Understandings, Searching, and Teachers) and Narayanasamy (24), the ASSET (Actioning Spirituality and Spiritual Care Education and Training in nursing) model. Both have been utilised to develop teaching and learning but these studies were limited by an exclusively Judaeo-Christian orientation and lacked adequate evaluation.

The TRUST model (22) for understanding spiritual care needs of patients is based upon experiential learning strategies and could be useful in teaching learners the importance of developing self-awareness and intentionality.

The ASSET (24) model emphasised the importance of self-awareness in nurses and patients for sustaining therapeutic relationships. This model embraces the entire nursing process from assessment to evaluation and elaborates upon competencies required to build and sustain the nurse-patient relationship on spiritual grounds.

Burkhart and Schmidt (25), drawing on Burkhart and Hogan's Spiritual Care in Nursing Practice theory (26), developed a Spiritual Care Educational and Reflective Program (SCERP), emphasising spiritual care-giving as an interactive discourse in nursing practice. They demonstrated that a combination of interactive and reflective practise was effective in developing learners' competence in understanding and approaching the spiritual care needs of patients and families. Burkhart and Schmidt (25) concluded that an integrated, process-oriented approach might be useful in teaching spiritual care.

Costello et al (27) investigated simulation as a teaching and learning method with respect to spiritual care. The simulation activity was effective as it allowed learners to practice therapeutic communication and use the nursing assessment process in given narrative scenarios focused on spiritual distress. The competencies showing improvement at a high level of significance included acknowledging spiritual needs of patients, making referrals, assessing spiritual needs and providing personal support and patient counselling. Learners also reported that discussing spirituality during the simulation session helped them to become more reflective in relating spiritual care to clinical scenarios.

Baldacchino (28) and Lemmer (29) attempted to develop awareness and facilitate spiritual care in nurses and other health care professionals. They used a variety of approaches including transcultural, religious, ethical and teaching methods. Compassionate care and empathetic communication were used to address spiritual care needs. Individual study, utilising a workbook with a supplemental DVD and self-reporting assessment, was found by Taylor et al (30) to be a useful strategy for students to develop understanding about their own spirituality and awareness of the spiritual care needs of their patients.

However, without an effective, educationally sound curriculum framework these innovative, creative strategies are disparate and fragmented in approach.

Developing Capability and Self-Determined Learning: A Solution?

The fragmented nature of spirituality within curricula inhibits the sharing and utilisation of good, effective and educationally sound approaches and methods such as those discussed above (22,23,27,29).

An effective way to promote successful curricula is to adopt and engage with Barnett's (31,32) concept of a tripartite model, incorporating, societal, institutional and learner's needs contributing to the development of competence and capability in knowledge, skills and attitudes. Capability goes beyond competency and involves learners having confidence in their competency and being able to apply it in a variety of settings. A holistic, learner-centred self-determined approach to curriculum is needed, involving an expansion and re-interpretation of principles of adult learning (andragogy). A shift in thinking towards self-determined learning and capability as well as competency (heutagogy) will enable the learner to develop space, promoting the learner as an 'architect' of learning. Reflective learning and workplace-based learning lend themselves to this approach. The tripartite model requires society to place due emphasis upon the integration and development of spirituality within the curriculum and learning institutes to facilitate students in the development of spiritual competence and capability.

The higher education environment stimulates learning through various systems and structures and these determine, when, how and what is learned within the curricula accepting that a curriculum is the total learning experience of individuals, not only within the learning institution but also within society and communities. These systems can either promote or inhibit the choice of what is learned and what skills are developed; clearly, over the past three decades the development of spirituality within the curriculum has been inhibited.

University education has traditionally been seen as a hierarchical relationship between the lecturer and the learner. The lecturer is viewed as the expert, who decides what the learner needs to know in terms of knowledge and skills and how they should be taught, which in turn is based upon the lecturer's competence and familiarity. This is especially so within nurse education that has been dominated by the apprentice and bio medical model influence upon the pedagogical process adopted within the curriculum. This can stifle creativity and fail to present a truly humanistic approach to a practice-orientated curriculum. There has been quiet revolution in educational methodologies (17,24), but current practice still reflects an hierarchical dyadic academic relationship. At its worst this can produce graduates who have not *learned how to learn* and therefore find it hard to adapt to a constantly changing professional world. Barnett (33) asserts that educators need 'to give serious attention to the potential for radical *educational innovation*' and be imaginative within their curricula (p.9), reflecting the passionate plea of McSherry and Draper (17) two decades earlier for curriculum innovation, and for educators to take a risk in developing creative approaches to these fundamental, complex concepts underpinning practice.

Barnett (34) alludes to a super complex changing world which presents 'proliferating and competing frameworks' of understanding (p.6). What constitutes learning, the development of knowledge, attitudes and skills in one context may not be appropriate for another context. Each, individual, group and community is unique; each is different in terms of perspective, values, need and demand for skills and knowledge. Curricula should reflect this diversity and adopt an approach that is learner-centric, avoiding the characteristic 'broad brush' approach to delivery that depersonalises learners who are exposed to predictable and fixed approaches to teaching and learning. However, Swinton and Pattison (35) suggest that the lack of conceptual clarity and diverse definitions that underpin the epistemological basis of spirituality provide a valuable opportunity for developing learning, and further suggest that the lack of clarity is a strength of this concept and can be used as a tool for developing holistic learning.

Embedding spirituality within the curriculum is complex. Barnett (31,32,34) provided guidance for educators developing complex curricula. He introduced the notion of a tripartite inter-dependent relationship between society, the learning institution and the student's needs. described above. Barnett (34) suggested that there is a temptation to view the relationship between knowledge and society in a binary form but 'that higher education, knowledge and society are mutually inter-dependent' (p.11), providing a guiding framework for the developing learning orientated curriculum, where knowledge is the product of the interaction of society and the university. If this interdependent relationship is not explored the curriculum will not be truly 'needs-led'. This raises three key questions: what are the knowledge, attitudes, skills and roles required to meet the demands of the groups or community served by the graduate; how is this to be determined and how are they to be prepared? In later works, Barnett and Coate (36) develop the notion of the tripartite relationship and the curriculum further, providing some guidance on how these questions can be addressed (Figure 5.1).

Whilst there is a clear association and interdependence of society, knowledge and higher education (31), the relationship is refined to such a level that determines what it is that a graduate needs to 'know' – (epistemological basis), how they need to act – (the skills required to fulfil the role) and what they need to 'become' (the ontological). Whilst these are functional domains, the emphasis is not upon what learners know, but their engagement with knowledge, that is 'knowing.' Equally, whilst 'acting' the skills may seem self-evident, the 'action domain can take on a pre-formative character' (36, p.105), especially where there has been little integration and the curriculum has been developed in a fragmented manner. The third domain, 'being' or attitude is, they suggest, typically the most neglected and yet paradoxically

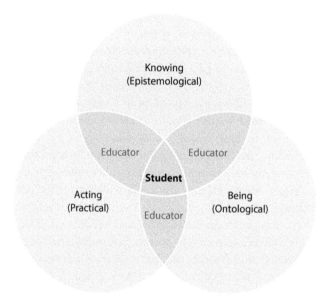

Figure 5.1 The concept of the tripartite relationship and the spiritual curriculum. (Adapted from Barnett R, Coate K, *Engaging the Curriculum in Higher Education*. Buckingham: SRHE and Open University Press; 2005.)

the most significant of the three domains, for without it, the others cannot function. Barnett and Coate (36) further suggest that 'being' in this context is related to the notion of 'self' and forms of knowing and acting in the world; that is, who we are, our attitudes and how we function, and is context specific. For example:

- **Knowing and Knowledge (Epistemological):** Spirituality in practice by exploring self and intentionality, including reflexivity and accepting the *Other*
- **Being and Attitude (Ontological):** Spiritual self-awareness and the use of self as an agency, including self-expression through creativity and inclusive expansion
- **Acting and Skill (Practical):** Quality assurance and improvement by creative encounters, including transformation and growth

In order to understand and translate curricula, the learner must have self-confidence and self-efficacy in the learning process; engagement with appropriate knowing and acting domains of the curricula driven by the learner will assist in the development of self, enabling a fully engaged learner (37). An adapted version of van Leeuwen and Cusveller's (38), spiritual competencies is presented in Chapter 1 of this book can be mapped onto Barnet and Coates' (36) domains. In order to develop this tripartite approach in the context of spiritually competent practice, each of these domains must be embedded within the curriculum.

Spiritual education clearly has three main components: Knowledge, Skill and Attitude. Though attitude traditionally refers to those behaviours congruent with professional values and standards, it could easily be seen as the ontological domain. Skills refer to those activities that enable learners to perform tasks effectively. Knowledge refers to the professional knowledge and evidence-based practice that allows the practitioner to act as a holistic practitioner. The three domains, together with their sub-components and characteristics, prepare the learner to practice with spiritual competence and capability. Spiritual education is not a passive education process, but an active and interactive one in which learners must get involved as whole people, as soul (ontology), body (skills) and mind (knowledge).

The concept of 'space' in terms of these three domains has been aptly explored by authors such as Barnett (32), where 'space' is described in both physical and educational terms. Physical space is that which can be seen, for example, within the built environment such as the lecture hall, refectory, classroom, off-campus buildings and study space; the non-built, such as the Virtual Learning Environment, internal and external structures, professional/vocational structures, books, course handbooks, peers, clubs and societies, etc. Learning within the pedagogical space; the epistemological space and the ontological space as Barnett (36) suggests 'Pedagogical space...includes not only epistemological space (the space to think the impossible), but ontological space, in which the learner can bring herself into a new state of being. The inspiring teacher, accordingly, gives the learner space in which she can become more fully herself, to gain her own air, to *become* ... [our emphasis] in an authentic way' (p.116). To develop and fully engage a learner it is essential that all the 'spaces' in which a learner learns are utilised. There are different kinds of learning spaces ... all have different educational emphases. However, whatever the 'space', it is full of messages, symbols and metaphors, and is never passive; it enables ways of seeing and becoming, whilst excluding others and promoting bias and influence. Maintaining authenticity within the curriculum, however, is challenging for curriculum planners; encouraging the learner to understand self and learn from within depends upon external agencies such as the Nursing and Midwifery Council (NMC), Quality Assurance Agency (QAA) and internal agencies such as regulatory and professional, and institutional features and values (43). However, we maintain that it is the role of the educator to enable learners to create, develop and utilise space effectively for their learning.

We can accept that learning takes place through the various systems and structures within the learning environment and these historically have largely determined, when, how and what is learned. These systems can either promote or inhibit the choice of what is learned and what skills are developed; in the case of spirituality this has been clearly stifled. However, distinctly we also learn within ourselves, within our own personal ontological space.

Rogers (39) suggests that learning is an innate process and the desire to learn is an internal process controlled by the learner him/herself, thus creating a personal ontological space. Consequently, within this personal ontological space, we learn from within ourselves and the teacher is viewed as a facilitator of learning. When something new is learned, our 'being,' that is the notion of who we are, is changed, as a new space, a new mode of being is created, and a new space of learning is entered (32) (see parallels with the psycho-spiritual frame of reference for occupational therapy discussed in Chapter 3). New learning possibilities are created, and the learner is encouraged and enabled to develop as an architect of learning, where learning is arranged around their activities and their real world experience rather than driven by pre-determined syllabi or curricula content. This enables what is to be learned to be context-specific, facilitating an authentic approach to learning. The learner then becomes a designer of learning, subsequently building an individual pattern of learning spaces and opportunities, drawing upon their own context-related technological, value-based, community, societal, subject and discipline knowledge and skills. The learner creates their own pattern of ideas and experiences relevant to their own mind, being and learning, embracing an holistic, authentic approach to learning. Key to this self-determined or heutagogical process of learning is the place of the learner – who is at the heart of the learning, it is the learner who drives what it is to be learned rather than the constraints of a prescribed syllabus or curriculum.

Barnett (33) suggests that there are a number of risks for adopting this approach to learning. In relation to the developing curriculum these can be associated with 'epistemological risk' – by following their interests, learning what they want to learn and creating their own curriculum, learners may end up with what he describes as a 'warped perspective or a skewed understanding of a field' (p.143). There is also a 'practical risk' – the learner may not have the practical skills to respond effectively to this learning approach, failing to develop and progress new skills. The pedagogical risk is concerned with developing a 'space-for-being' where the risk is 'ontological' shaping the learner's 'being' and subsequently their personal identity. This is the most significant risk and is ever present in the pedagogical processes that are employed in this approach. Nonetheless, it is this risk that promotes creativity and development of the curriculum

The risks can be managed and reduced by adoption of heutagogical principles. Heutagogy provides a framework for learning that harnesses and manages this dynamic and complex notion of learning, providing a curriculum approach that provides a 21st century approach to learning and teaching congruent with the demands of contemporary society. Heutagogy, as described by Hase and Kenyon (40) is an educational theory that facilitates self-determined learning, where participants are encouraged to research their learning and practice interests and base their learning on these interests and their aspirations. In this approach to learning the learner and their place in community and society becomes the fulcrum of learning. There is a philosophical shift away from pedagogy/andragogy where traditionally the learner was often a passive recipient of knowledge, where the lecturer/teacher adopted the role of knowledge expert who simply converted their knowledge, determining what was learned and how it was to be learned.

The origins of heutagogy (40) lie in complexity theory and capability development. It expands upon the concept of life-wide and life-long learning and harnesses self-determined learning. Hase and Kenyon (40) argue that there is an ever-increasing interdependency of events and that the ability to predict future events and authentic learning is becoming increasingly challenging. Consequently, learning is becoming much more emergent as a process and more natural, adaptive and realistic, with predictability and outcome much less certain. Complexity theory, coupled with the notion of capability described by Stephenson and Yorke (41), provides the process of acquiring not only skills and knowledge, but also the ethics and judgements required to solve unfamiliar problems in unfamiliar contexts. A capable individual, as opposed to a competent person who performs effectively in the present, is someone who is also forward-thinking and concerned with potential realisation, imaging the future and making it happen.

Learning is increasingly concerned with what we do, and the development of those key skills and abilities appropriate for the changing, dynamic and contested work place and contemporary society. It is clear spirituality is part of what people do.

Heutagogy draws upon the key perspectives offered by Stephenson and Yorke (41), Argyryris and Schon (42), Knowles (43), Carr and Kemmis (44) and Lave and Wenger (45) in an attempt to develop an holistic approach to learning, developing independent capability and the capacity to question self, values and assumptions (46). Heutagogy is prospective in approach, enabling the development of community-led knowledge, skills and attitudes especially suited to forming capability in the application of complex concepts such as spirituality.

Heideggerian in perspective, heutagogy asserts that people make sense of the world around them, generalise from their perceptions, conceptualise and perceive invariances. People consequently have the potential to learn continuously and in real time by interacting with their environment. They learn throughout their life span, leading to ideas rather than the force-fed knowledge of others. They enhance their creativity and develop intuitive skills. Intuition is an integral part of the heutagogical learning process, drawing upon reflective and double-loop learning – it includes aspects of action and reflective learning, valuing experience and interaction, but importantly it draws heavily upon community-based and societal-based learning. This is an approach that responds to the challenge of enabling the development of people who can cope with a rapidly changing world, and places great emphasis upon holism, self, capability, community, needs of society and a focus upon learning as opposed to teaching (37).

Bhoyrub et al (47), examining the notion of heutagogy and its relevance to nurse education, assert that health care training and education becomes increasingly complex due to the multi-faceted nature of health care management and delivery. Heutagogy provides 'a potential-packed approach to clinical learning that provides an alternative lens from which to both view and construct practice-based educational components' of courses (p.326); it is this alternative lens that is required to present an informed spiritual curriculum, consequently presenting a creative, pedagogical-based approach to developing spiritual competence in practitioners.

Two such methods that are consistent with a heutagogical approach to learning are solution-focused learning and mentor-assisted learning.

Solution-Focused Teaching and Learning

Solution-focused teaching and learning can be described as a transformative learning and teaching experience (48,49). It is a method that activates learners to become committed, engaged citizens, and to recognise that learning and development requires change to take place at individual, societal and cultural levels. Solution-focused approaches to teaching and learning are concerned with constructing solutions rather than dwelling on problems; it is consequently an approach that looks forward, towards solutions, rather than backwards, by studying problems. It is a transformative learning experience that builds upon those features based upon the discovery of challenging beliefs, values and solutions. It is an approach that develops critical consciousness, collective identity, and develops solution-orientated strategies for change. It develops the cognitive and affective domain of participants and conscious competence in skill development. Adopting a real-world approach to teaching and learning, it encourages teaching and learning that focuses upon strengths, abilities and hopes, and distinctly encourages thinking in terms of possibilities. It provides a developmental framework that would enable models and strategies illustrated by Narayanasamy (5), Cone and Giske (23), Barss (22), Burkhart and Schmidt (25) and Costello et al (27) to be used effectively within the curriculum, providing a firm pedagogical basis for their development.

Successful Solution-focused teaching strategies include authentic work-based learning, mentor-assisted learning, peer mentorship, case study examination, role-play, simulation and rehearsal. Scaffolding and the use of complex solution-focused exercises, situated context activities, community-based and cross-disciplinary learning and solution pursuit exercises all come under this rubric, used as a learner- and community-based learning approach. Solution-focused teaching and learning offer a model of collective cohesiveness, enabling the development of capability that has a robust pedagogical basis.

Mentoring and Heutagogy

Mentoring is an intervention that supports those individuals with less experience within any given context in their personal, social and professional development. However, this somewhat simplistic description fails to reflect the multifaceted and complex nature of the mentoring relationship. Defining mentorship is complex, due in part to the multidimensional nature of the role. There have been many attempts to define mentorship in a precise way. However, it is recognised that definitions, and consequently the role of the mentor, should reflect the social context of implementation.

The mentoring process is often associated with social developments, as individuals pass through their various life transitions and stages. Learning and personal development are fundamental to this process, and the UK apprenticeship style of learning has strong connections with mentoring. Roberts (50) offers an all-embracing definition of mentoring that reflects this view:

> … a supportive process; a supportive relationship; a helping process; a teaching learning process; a reflective process; a career development process; a formalised process and a role constructed by or for the mentor. The contingent attributes of the mentoring phenomena appear as coaching, sponsoring, role modelling, assessing and informal process. (p.162)

It is not the aim of this chapter to explore in detail the many attempts to define the mentor. It is clear when reviewing the literature that there are two commonly occurring facets: relationship and reciprocity. Mentoring will be based upon a relationship; this can be either within a dyad or between one mentor and a group of mentees. Reciprocity is where an exchange element exists between the people involved in the relationship. Mentoring is a term which is used interchangeably and is not consistent across studies or within practice (51,52), and is compounded by the observation that the length of the relationship is not consistent – it may or may not be predetermined. Recently, the UK has seen higher education institutions adopting a different approach to mentoring. Peer mentoring has emerged as a strategy to enhance development and retention and ease the transition of learners into university. Whilst Andrews and Clarke (52) allude to the complexities of defining the peer mentor, Lennox Terrion and Leonard (51) provide a useful definition of the *peer mentor* as a person who provides an assistive relationship in which two (or more) individuals of similar age/or experience work together, either informally or formally, to fulfil some kind of informational and/or emotional need (p.150). This moves away from the hierarchical nature of the relationship that underpins traditional mentoring. Whilst the peer mentor still holds a higher level of experience and knowledge than the mentee, they are typically more approachable, find it easier to empathise, and have a greater ability to provide psycho-social and task-orientated support.

It is widely accepted that mentoring enhances the learning experience for all participants, and existing literature suggests (52,53) there is little doubt that peer mentorship will contribute positively to the undergraduate's experience in higher education.

Crucially, the mentor enables the mentee to engage in the academic community faster and more efficiently. This process of becoming a participant in the community is viewed very much as a socio-cultural process in the acquisition of new knowledge and skills (53). Thus, learning is equated with the process in which participation moulds knowledge and identity.

Learning is a social and situated process where the development of skill, knowledge and understanding are grounded within the institutional environment where learners interact within various processes of participation and engagement. Alred and Garvey (54) appraise the literature concerning mentoring in the context of knowledge productivity and introduce the notion of the 'learning landscape' to illustrate the shift from apprentice type instructor-led learning to a much more social and holistic model of learning with the learner at the centre of the process. They allude to the value of mentorship within learning, and give emphasis to placing the learner at the heart of an authentic learning process. This places emphasis upon the role of engagement described by Lave and Wenger (45) and the notion of 'situated learning.' Lave and Wenger assert that learning is socially constructed but distinctly takes place within an authentic context. As learners engage in authentic discussion and activities over a period of time, a community of practice is formed where the learner is fully engaged with the practice of the community. Mentor-assisted learning used alongside solution-focused approaches to teaching and learning provides an exceptionally powerful tool for learning.

Alred and Garvey (54) introduce the notion of the 'learning landscape' as a scaffold to illustrate the context of knowledge productivity within a community. This scaffold represents the social and cultural influences that shape the learner, and illustrates the shift to a social and holistic model of the learning landscape that is driven by the learner. They identified seven key areas (54) as part of the learning landscape having particular relevance to the mentoring relationship in this setting:

- The acquisition of subject matter expertise and skill directly related to the scope of target competence.
- Learning to solve problems by using domain specific expertise.
- Developing reflective and critical thinking skills conducive to locating paths leading to new knowledge and its application.
- Securing communication skills that provide access to the knowledge network of others and those that enrich the learning environment.
- Procuring skills that regulate motivation and affections related to learning.
- Promoting stability to enable specialisation, cohesion and integration.
- Causing creative turmoil to instigate improvement and innovation. (p.264)

In order for this landscape to succeed in developing spiritual competence and capability, the learner needs to be at the centre of the learning process and engaged within the community. Learning within and as a consequence the mentoring relationship enables the process of knowledge production in the learner to be enhanced. The peer mentor aids and facilitates this learning, enabling the mentee to participate in academic life much earlier, choosing and attaining the 'subject matter expertise and skill and in developing reflective and critical thinking skills conducive to new knowledge' (p.264). The relationship between the mentor and the mentee contributes to breaking down some of the barriers that inhibit participation, thus enabling the mentee to rapidly access the support mechanisms available and engage with academic activities and securing communication skills that provide access to the knowledge of others, challenging the traditional role of the lecturer as the expert in knowledge.

It is when considering the notion of 'inside knowledge' – the knowledge that is generated from someone's experience – that the real impact upon learning begins to materialise. Stringer-Cawyer, Simonds and Davis (55) suggest that the process of mentoring facilitates socialisation, as mentees learn and adapt to the processes, values and social knowledge available within the community. Early access to this inside knowledge would help the learner to learn more effectively to establish a stronger sense of belonging and participation within the learning community. It would also aid the development of confidence in selecting learning experiences. The peer mentor, by virtue of their 'inside knowledge', drawing upon their experiences, is able to translate the curriculum, socially constructing and offering guidance in choosing what and how to learn, and how to utilise the learning for development of skills and attitudes in practice.

The basis of Lave and Wenger's (46) assertion concerning knowledge productivity is rooted in their observation that learning is viewed as a form of participation and that the learner should be at the centre of the learning process. The central tenet of 'situated learning' is that learning, and the production of knowledge, is generated by the experience. Thus learning is equated with the process by which participation moulds knowledge and identity. It is participation, facilitated by the peer mentor in this community, that enables, in part, the mentee to access inside knowledge. Alred and Garvey (54) suggest that it is this engagement with the learning process that gives impetus to the value of informal situated learning, and within this context 'a mentor encourages persistence and effort' (p.267). One way of doing this is by helping the mentee focus on the process of learning and on progress made rather than on their ability to do the tasks in hand, adopting Hase and Kenyon's (40) approach to self-determined learning.

Self-efficacy is essential for learner success in this context. The belief that one can succeed is clearly linked to positive performance. Bandura and Locke (56) emphasise the importance of self-efficacy: 'Self-efficacy beliefs ... affect whether individuals think in self-enhancing or self-debilitating ways' (p.87). Embracing a culture of confidence, reassurance and success aids successful learning. Margolis (57) suggested that self-efficacy was essential and those learners with strong self-efficacy are characterised by higher motivation, greater effort, and greater persistence. Consequently, they achieve more. Roberts (58) also suggested, in relation to self-efficacy, that the mentor enabled the mentee to discover latent abilities. The process also encouraged growth in confidence, personal growth, increased awareness, increased effectiveness and self-actualisation. The mentor provides a model of positive behaviour that reflects success and experience, acting as a powerful transmitter of values and attitudes, which reinforce successful learning. Mentors contributed to 'self–efficacy' by procuring skills that Alred and Garvey (54) suggest enhance learning and the production of knowledge.

Engagement with the process of mentoring within the context of learning enables the learner to rapidly inhabit and navigate the systems, structures and spaces within the learning environment but also provides access to the inside knowledge that the mentor has developed. The mentor helps translate reality, and supports the mentee in inhabiting their own internalised patterns of reasoning, facilitating the development of a learning landscape and space to learn. The peer mentor is able to facilitate co-reflection, enabling the mentee to articulate what they did, their learning and knowledge preferences and how these can be interpreted, constructed and applied within the real world. For this landscape to succeed in knowledge and skill acquisition, the learner needs to be at the centre of this process and engaged within the community. It is this process that learning as part of a mentoring relationship that enables the skills, knowledge and role of the individual to be enhanced. This represents the social and cultural influences that shape the learner, and illustrates the shift to a social and holistic model of learning.

Conclusion

A shift in thinking and practice towards heutagogy will enable the learner, with the support of mentor-assisted learning and a solution-focused approach, to develop space. The learner becomes an architect of their own learning and mentoring enables learners to learn about the nature of understanding and their role in making knowledge, inspiring them to develop their spiritual practice. We do not advocate that learners are given a 'tabula rasa' on entry to learning within a curriculum, as this is unlikely to provide the response health care professions demand. Indeed, Canning and Callan (59) suggest that there are two prerequisites for an heutagogical approach: 'emotional literacy and emotional identity' (p.76) both of which, we suggest, are developed in learners who have experienced effective mentorship within this approach to learning.

We propose that the adoption of heutagogical principles, and Barnett and Coates (36) tripartite curriculum, respond to the challenge set by McSherry and Draper (17) and Lewinson et al (10). Heutagogy is an approach that can enhance the curriculum and learning opportunities around spiritually competent and capable practice. This framework, drawing upon mentor-assisted learning and solution-focused teaching and learning, provides a way for educators to embed spirituality in practice.

References

1. Royal College of Nursing. Spirituality in nursing care. 2015. Available at: http://www.rcn.org.uk/development/practice/spirituality/about_spirituality_in_nursing_care (accessed 4/3/16).
2. NANDA International. *Nursing Diagnoses: Definitions & Classification 2015–2017* (10th edition). Herdman THH, Kamitsuru S (eds). Wiley-Blackwell; 2014.
3. Ali G, Wattis J, Snowden M. Why are spiritual aspects of care so hard to address in nursing education?' A literature review (1993–2015). *International Journal of Multidisciplinary Comparative Studies.* 2015; 2(1):7–31.
4. Chilman AM, Thomas M. *Understanding Nursing Care.* London: Churchill Livingstone; 1988.
5. Narayanasamy A. Nurses' awareness and preparedness in meeting their patients' spiritual needs. *Nurse Education Today.* 1993; 13:196–201.
6. Baldacchino DR. Teaching on the spiritual dimension in care: the perceived Impact on undergraduate nursing learners. *Nurse Education Today.* 2008; 28:501–512.
7. Benner P, Sutphen M, Leonard V, Day L. *Educating Nurses: A Call for Radical Transformation.* Chichester, UK: Jossey-Bass/Carnegie Foundation for the Advancement of Teaching; 2010.
8. McSherry W, Jamieson S. Nurses knowledge and attitudes, an online survey of nurses' perceptions of spirituality and spiritual care. *Journal of Clinical Nursing.* 2011; 20:1757–1767.
9. Ross L, van Leeuwen R, Baldacchino D, Giske T, McSherry W, Narayanasamy A, Downes C, Jarvis P, Schep-Akkerman A. Learner nurses perceptions of spirituality and competence in delivering spiritual care: a European pilot study. *Nurse Education Today.* 2014; 34(5):697–702.
10. Lewinson LP, McSherry W, Kevern P. Spirituality in pre-registration nurse education and practice: a review of the literature. *Nurse Education Today.* 2015; 36:806–814.
11. Timmins F, et al. An exploration of the extent of inclusion of spirituality and spiritual care concepts in core nursing textbooks. *Nurse Education Today.* 2014. Available at: http://dx.doi.org/10.1016/j.nedt.2014.05.008 (accessed 13/12/14).
12. McSherry W, Cash K. The language of spirituality: an emerging taxonomy. *International Journal of Nursing Studies.* 2004; 41:151–161.
13. Prentis S, Rogers M, Wattis J, Jones J, Stephenson J. Healthcare lecturers' perceptions of spirituality in education. *Nursing Standard.* 2014; 29(3):44–52
14. Nursing and Midwifery Council. The code: professional standards of practice and behaviour for nurses and midwives. 2015. Available at: http://www.nmc-uk.org/The-revised-Code/The-revised-Codein-full/ (accessed 3/4/16).
15. Yilmaz M, Gurler H. The efficacy of integrating spirituality into undergraduate nursing curricula. *Nursing Ethics.* 2014; 21(8):929–945.
16. General Medical Council. Good medical practice: working with doctors working for patients. 2013. Available at: http://www.gmc-uk.org/static/documents/content/GMP_.pdf (accessed 30/6/16).

17. McSherry W, Draper P. The spiritual dimension: why the absences within nursing curricula. *Nurse Education Today.* 1997; 17:413–417.
18. Cockell N, McSherry W. Spiritual care in nursing: an overview of published international research. *Journal of Nursing Management.* 2012; 20:958–969.
19. Palmer PJ. Teaching with heart and soul: reflections on spirituality in teacher education. *Journal of Teacher Education.* 2003; 54(5):376–385.
20. Cotton S, Zebracki K, Rosenthal SL, Tsevat J, Drotar D. Religion/spirituality and adolescent health outcomes: a review. *Journal of Adolescent Health.* 2006; 38:472–480.
21. Cooper K, Chang E, Sheehan A, Johnson A. The impact of spiritual care education upon preparing undergraduate nursing learners to provide spiritual care. *Nurse Education Today.* 2013; 33:1057–1061.
22. Barss K. Building bridges: an interpretive phenomenological analysis of nurse educators' clinical experience using the T.R.U.S.T. model of inclusive spiritual care. *International Journal of Nurse Education Scholarship.* 2012; 9:1–15.
23. Cone P, Giske T. Teaching spiritual care - a grounded theory study among undergraduate nursing educators. *Journal of Clinical Nursing.* 2012; 22:1951–1960.
24. Narayanasamy A. ASSET: a model for actioning spirituality and spiritual care education and training in nursing. *Nurse Education Today.* 1999; 19:274–285.
25. Burkhart L, Schmidt W. Measuring effectiveness of a spiritual care pedagogy in nursing education. *Journal of Professional Nursing.* 2012; 28:315–321.
26. Burkhart L, Hogan N. An experiential theory of spiritual care in nursing practice. *Qualitative Health Research.* 2008; 18:928–938.
27. Costello M. Atinaja-Galler J, Hedberg M. The use of simulation to instruct learners on the provision of spiritual care - a pilot study. *Journal of Holistic Nursing American Holistic Nurses Association.* 2012; 30:4.
28. Baldacchino DR. Teaching on the spiritual dimension in care: the perceived impact on qualified nurses. *Nurse Education and Practice.* 2010; 11:47–53.
29. Lemmer C. Reflections on teaching spirituality in the healthcare environment. *Journal of Holistic Nursing.* 2010; (2):145–9.
30. Taylor EJ, Mamier I, Bhjri K, Anton T, Peterson F. Efficacy of a self-study programme to teach spiritual care. *Journal of Clinical Nursing.* 2009; 18:1131–1140.
31. Barnett R. *The Limits of Competence: Knowledge, Higher Education and Society.* Buckingham: SRHE, Open University Press; 1994
32. Barnett R. Knowing and becoming in the higher education curriculum. *Studies in Higher Education.* 2010; 34(4):429–440.
33. Barnett R. *Conditions of Flexibility: Securing a More Responsive Higher Education System.* York, UK: Higher Education Academy; 2014.
34. Barnett R. Learning about learning: a conundrum and a possible resolution. *London Review of Education.* 2011; 9(1):5–13.
35. Swinton J, Pattison S. Moving beyond clarity: towards a thin, vague, and useful understanding of spirituality in nursing care. *Nursing Philosophy.* 2010; 11 (4):226–237
36. Barnett R, Coate K. *Engaging the Curriculum in Higher Education.* Buckingham: SRHE and Open University Press; 2005.

37. Snowden M, Halsall J. Community development: a shift in thinking towards heutagogy. *International Journal of Multi-Disciplinary Comparative Studies*. 2014; 1(3):81–91.

38. van Leeuwen R, Cusveller B. Nursing competencies for spiritual care. *Journal of Advanced Nursing*. 2004; 48(3):234–246

39. Rogers C. *Client-Centred Therapy: Its Current Practice, Implications and Theory*. London: Constable; 1951.

40. Hase S, Kenyon C. *Self Determined Learning: Heutagogy in Action*. London: Bloomsbury; 2013.

41. Stephenson J, Yorke M (eds). *Capability and Quality in Higher Education. (Teaching and Learning in Higher Education)*. London: Kogan Page; 1998.

42. Argyryris C, Schon DA. *Theory in Practice: Increasing Professional Effectiveness*. San Francisco, CA: Jossey Bass; 1974.

43. Knowles, M. *Self-Directed Learning: A guide for Learners and Teachers*. Cambridge: Cambridge Adult Education; 1983.

44. Carr W, Kemmis S. *Becoming Critical: Education Knowledge and Action Research*. Geelong: Deakin University Press; 1986.

45. Lave J, Wenger E. *Situated Learning: Legitimate Peripheral Participation*. New York: Cambridge University Press; 1991.

46. Canning N, Callan S. Heutagogy: spirals of reflection to empower learners in higher education. *Reflective Practice*. 2010; 11(1):71–82.

47. Bhoyrub J, Hurley J, Neilson GR, Ramsay M, Smith M. Practice based learning approach. *Nurse Education in Practice*. 2010; 19(6):322–326.

48. McAllister M. Doing practice differently: solution focused nursing. *Journal of Advanced Nursing*. 2003; 41(6):528–535.

49. Mezirow J. *Learning as Transformation*. San Francisco: Jossey-Bass; 2000.

50. Roberts A. Mentoring revisited: a phenomenological reading of the literature. *Mentoring & Tutoring*. 2000; 8(2):145–170.

51. Lennox Terrion J, Leonard D. A taxonomy of the characteristics of learner peer mentors in higher education: findings from a literature review. *Mentoring & Tutoring*. 2007; 15(2):149–164

52. Andrews J, Clark R. *Peer Mentoring Works! How Peer Mentoring Enhances Learner Success in Higher Education*. Birmingham: Aston University; 2011.

53. Snowden M, Hardy T. Peer Mentorship: Yes! It Does Have a Positive Effect on Learner Retention and Academic Success for Both Mentor and Mentee. *Journal of Widening Participation and Lifelong Learning*. 2012; 14:76–92.

54. Alred G, Garvey B. Learning to produce knowledge – the contribution of mentoring. *Mentoring & Tutoring*. 2000; 8(3):261–277.

55. Stringer-Cawyer C, Simonds C, Davis S. Mentoring to facilitate socialisation: the case of the new faculty member. *Qualitative Studies in Higher Education*. 2002; 15(2):225–242.

56. Bandura A, Locke EA. Negative self-efficacy and goal effects revisited. *Journal of Applied Psychology*. 2003; 88:87–99.

57. Margolis H. Increasing struggling learner's self-efficacy: what tutors can do and say. *Mentoring & Tutoring*. 2005; 13(2):221–238.

58. Roberts A. Mentoring revisited: a phenomenological reading of the literature. *Mentoring & Tutoring*. 2000; 8(2):145–170.

59. Canning N, Callan S. Heutagogy: spirals of reflection to empower learners in higher education. *Reflective Practice*. 2010; 11(1):71–82.

Supporting the Practitioner 6

Martin Seager and Mike Bush

Introduction

This chapter is based on over 60 years of combined experience, practice and research within the NHS, Social Services and the voluntary sector that we have accumulated between us. Mike has a background in social work and Martin has a background in psychology. Our mutual passion for preventing suicide initially brought us together several years ago and has led us increasingly into collaborative efforts to make a difference to the quality and accessibility of care in our society. This has for us highlighted the enormous gap in theory and practice relating to how we care for the practitioners whose job it is to provide care. We have between us written extensively on this subject and run numerous teaching events, training workshops and conferences. In this chapter we attempt to make a common-sense argument for caring for the hearts and minds of society's care workers based upon a framework that honours the personal and the spiritual aspects of humanity as a core part of science.

Mind-Blindness: Bad Science And Worse Philosophy

In the West, since the age of enlightenment we have taken an increasingly secular and materialistic view of the universe which subordinates mind to matter and splits mind from body. This is bad science and leads to false assumptions that the physical brain is the objective source of all our mental experience and that the subjective mind by definition is something illusory or biased which needs to be factored out of science (1). Where mind goes, there follows spirit and anything spiritual is also seen in the West as unscientific. Indeed, within traditional Western science, spirituality and competence are not generally viewed as compatible concepts and so the very title of this book may induce a classification in bookshops that ranks alongside astrology and fortune-telling.

However, even physicists, for example Capra (2), are increasingly recognising that mind is in fact at the root of all scientific observation and theory. There is no mind-free observation and we have to include the dimension of the mind and spirit in any scientific model of the universe. In Eastern traditions there is already a greater awareness that knowledge of the universe and enlightenment can only be obtained from the inside out, not the outside in. We are part of the universe, not bystanders. Such a perspective is crucial if we are ever to be properly scientific about the intersubjective ('mind to mind') and relational processes that we call 'care'.

Care, Science and the Human Spirit

Good quality care must have a spiritual element. It ultimately involves a meeting *between* minds where someone in need feels a connection with someone else who has the resources to attend to that need as a fellow human being. In traditional medicalised mental health science this is often mistakenly called a 'placebo' or a 'non-specific' effect but in psychological and spiritual terms this human connection is in truth a primary effect and a core aspect of all healing.

As Carl Rogers (3,4) demonstrated in his research decades ago, to be cared for successfully is by definition an *interpersonal* matter that involves *empathy*, *warmth* and *genuineness*. These vital human qualities can only be measured subjectively in our hearts and minds. From childhood onwards, human beings can quickly recognise when they are genuinely cared about and cared for. Empathy, warmth and genuineness are the easiest things to measure subjectively but in a scientific and policy framework that only values objective numerical values and outcomes, the spiritual essence of care can get completely lost, dishonoured and even violated.

However, even in traditional scientific studies all the clues are there. In particular, all psychotherapy outcome studies when taken collectively show the big picture that it is 'relationship factors' rather than therapy techniques or models that account for the bulk of the variance in outcomes (5). We also know that love and care are not simply 'soft' phenomena. The scientific evidence shows that love shapes even our brains and physical development (6). However, even when faced with these findings, rather than focussing on better understanding of these ancient and universal relationship factors, Western therapy research persists in looking for new and better 'objective' care techniques. This means that when it comes to the humanity of our public care services, our energies are going into examining behavioural technicalities rather than patterns of connection between the hearts, minds and souls of individuals (7). Of course, if there were no difference between these two levels it would be impossible for human beings to act, pretend, lie or be insincere. Care only works when it is sincere and sincerity can only be measured at the level of the heart and mind.

Contemporary Western health and social care science remains fixated on developing new clinical techniques of care rather than on illuminating the transformative human psychological and spiritual qualities that have been helping and healing people in all cultures since time immemorial. It is perhaps not surprising therefore that we have now entered an age of increased personal and spiritual burn-out where, over and above financial constraints and staff shortages, care professionals are being expected to function like robots, delivering manualised techniques according to prescribed methods and being measured less in terms of quality of care and more in terms of quantitative and financial targets. In the

West, even an initiative such as 'mindfulness' (8) which is aimed perhaps at injecting more spirituality into our care systems is in danger of becoming yet another manualised and prescriptive approach.

If care is personal but care science is depersonalised, it is clear that there will be a philosophical and cultural rift in providing care models that fully embrace what it means to be human. If the relationship between care provider and care recipient is being neglected, how much more is the relationship between the care provider and those on whom he or she depends for support and nurturance? In this chapter we examine the vital question of the care, support and back-up that the carer also needs if the caring role is to be sustainable and satisfying. We argue that care cannot be spiritually competent unless the spiritual energies of the carer are also continuously supported and refreshed. This means having a model of care that includes the relationship between the carer and the supportive environment. The spirituality of care can then be seen as not just an individual or *intra*personal phenomenon but also as an *inter*personal, systemic and dynamic one.

The Psychological and Spiritual Needs of the Care Provider

The 'Carer Care' or ABC Model

The two of us (9,10) advocate a 'carer care' or 'A × B × C' model of care in which the emotional and spiritual needs of the carer for support (C) must be factored in to the caring process to energise the primary relationship between the carer (A) and the recipient of care (B). In common sense terms this means that care can only be as good as the mental state of the carer and the mental state of the carer depends in turn on the support and nutrition of the working environment.

All of us when in need of care have the right to encounter a care provider whose mind is in a receptive and energised state to attend to our needs. However, these emotional resources for care are not usually prioritised in any traditional list of health care competencies. Whilst there are stringent codes of conduct for care professionals set both by their professional and employing organisations, there are no similarly enshrined written codes relating to the quality of support that care providers themselves are entitled to if they are to avoid losing the energy to care through overwhelming stress, compassion fatigue and burn-out. This is in some ways strange given the unarguably high levels of stress, burn-out, sickness and absence that we find in the public care sector. For example, staff ill health costs £45m per annum in the social care sector alone (10).

Health care is seen primarily as a fixed skill or competence rather than as a dynamic process that requires emotional and spiritual nutrition and there is a mind-blindness to the needs of the caring mind. Indeed, whenever the well-being of care providers is written about, it is usually only in terms of *self*-care, indicating a belief that professional care workers are expected to dig deep within and find yet more energy to self-care on top of caring for their clients and patients.

We argue that emphasising only self-care in those who are already caring for others is missing the point in terms of generating the mental and spiritual energy that is required for care and compassion. Human beings cannot simply create their own spiritual energy from a vacuum. They need nurturing relationships with other people and outside sources so that their own energy can be constantly replenished. For this to happen, the needs of care-givers have to be recognised and the working environment has to be designed to meet those needs.

What sustains and what depletes the spirit and morale of care workers?

Once this question is asked, it is not so hard to answer. The problem is that the question is not asked often enough because the morale and spiritual energy of care workers is not sufficiently acknowledged to be a major mediating factor in the quality of care. Quality of care is usually perceived to come primarily from training in skills, techniques and competencies. The morale and spiritual state of those providing care is often regarded merely as a background factor or simply overlooked. This means that conceptualising the 'competence' of care as incorporating a spiritual dimension involves a major paradigm-shift. It is time to fully recognise that the human spirit needs to be factored into the science of health care, not factored out as a 'non-specific' variable. This is essentially the point behind the excellent concept of 'intelligent kindness' articulated by John Ballatt and Penelope Campling in their book of the same name (11). These authors, who both have an NHS background, argue that humanising the culture of our public health care, including for those who work in it, is vital if the whole enterprise is to become liberating and successful rather than oppressive and dysfunctional. They outline the unintended human consequences of a politically and financially driven performance management culture obsessed with organisational restructuring. They also look at ways of restoring the heart and soul of public care services through reclaiming the ancient and public-spirited concept of *kindness*.

Similarly, Stephen Wright (12) calls burn-out a 'spiritual crisis' and outlines the factors that he believes cause burn-out and those that prevent it. Wright makes a clear distinction between burn-out and stress. He emphasises that stress is a more specific and transient phenomenon whereas burn-out is a more lasting state of spiritual depletion and a defensive shutdown that develops cumulatively when daily stresses are built up without being relieved or attended to. Burn-out manifests itself in numbness, detachment and disengagement, in many ways like a kind of 'depression'. Wright makes it clear that at the root of spiritual burn-out is a spiritual disconnection from self, from others and from sources of meaning. This conception of burn-out also fits very well with the findings of Menzies-Lyth (13), who showed how nursing care systems in general hospitals can quickly become defensive and depersonalised to avoid overwhelming anxiety and distress in staff. The danger of burn-out for all concerned can be seen very powerfully in Dobbin's report on General Practitioners (14):

> The measure of burn-out that impacted most on the patient satisfaction was depersonalisation, described as an 'unfeeling or impersonal response toward recipients of one's service, care, treatment or instruction'. That is about as close a description of a lack of compassion that I can think of. You cut yourself off from understanding your patient's viewpoint, from empathising with their position, mirroring their circumstances emotionally.

Seager et al (2007) (cited in [1]) list the top five universal psychological and spiritual needs of the human condition, which can be simplified as follows:

1. To be loved
2. To be heard
3. To belong
4. To make a difference
5. To have meaning and purpose

These universal needs apply equally to all of us whether we are giving care or receiving it. As carers we cannot sustain the caring role if our own human needs too are not met within our working environment. Mike, in his workshops on looking after care practitioners, regularly states that 'we cannot deliver any hardware if we do not at the same time look after the software'. Martin argues that emotional nutrition, like physical nutrition, is vital in maintaining a 'receptive' state of mind that is needed to care for others. Without emotional nutrition there will be emotional toxicity and emotional depletion (9). According to this view, even in an environment filled with good intentions, emotional toxicity and depletion result from an unhealthy ratio between emotional burden and support or between emotional expenditure and input. Martin outlines three domains that influence the spiritual energy levels of care givers: (a) capacity factors, (b) burden factors and (c) support factors (see more below).

The act of caring in itself carries a necessary emotional cost. Psychologically, caring for others means identifying with pain and suffering, and this means willingly entering difficult emotional spaces. Caring for another cannot work in relieving pain unless the person being cared for can see an impact on the carer. Seeing that one's suffering affects another is the very psychological and spiritual basis of change and transformation in suffering. Touching and being touched by the heart and mind of another creates the spiritual connection that enables relief and comfort. This happens from the cradle to the grave as all of us seek recognition and understanding in the responses of others.

Of course, there can therefore be an intrinsic value and meaning in caring for others which feeds the spiritual resources of the carer. However, identifying with suffering and entering difficult emotional spaces is draining and can be toxic, especially if those spaces are traumatic. This means that if there is no thought given to how the spiritual and emotional cost of care will be compensated for and replenished, any care-giving individual or system is at constant risk of breakdown.

Mike's Story – A Personal Illustration of a Broken Carer

The following personal story from one of us (Mike) shows just how badly things can go wrong for a professional care-worker when working in an environment that is spiritually toxic and lacking in emotional nutrition.

> More than 40 years ago I trained to do a very demanding, stressful job as a social worker. During my training, there was nothing taught on the course relating to the importance of looking after ourselves. All the emphasis was on understanding and meeting the needs of service users and carers and, although this is our raison d'être, it is all too easy to forget about our own needs in the pressure to meet the needs of others. To do so can lead to drastic consequences.
>
> In 2000 I suffered a very severe mental breakdown due to an intolerable combination of extremely stressful work-related pressures, problems and a bullying boss. I felt like a dead man walking. My body was still working but there was no one at the controls anymore. It was an abrupt change – one moment I was a senior mental health social worker, a very busy, 'together' professional, and the next I was designated a mental health service user, feeling utterly useless, extremely vulnerable, powerless and terrified.

This year of living hell launched me on a journey of understanding and taught me so many things about severe mental distress. Among the lessons I learned in the hardest possible way was the great importance of understanding and looking after my own mental health. This led me to develop a teaching session on strategies for promoting and protecting the mental health of social workers, which I have been teaching for the last 10 years at universities in the Yorkshire area.

I am told by senior social work lecturers that my sessions have been highly evaluated and valued by students. I asked some students in the third year of their course if they had done anything on this subject before; I was astonished to find they had not. I asked myself why and came to the conclusion that it's so obvious it gets missed.

There are some fundamental lessons here for social workers around recognizing your own humanity. We are not a separate species to service users and carers. A social work degree is not a suit of armour. Cut us and we do in fact bleed. Together with this we need to recognize our own needs, review these and have a care plan for ourselves. Even the toughest, most resilient people can have mental health and other problems that, if not accepted and dealt with, will lead to breaking point. Is prevention not better than cure?

Sadly I am not the first social worker to have had a breakdown. This also applies to people in other caring professions, who also do difficult demanding stressful work.

Based on these personal experiences of breakdown and of teaching others about how to protect the mental and spiritual well-being of social workers, Mike has launched a campaign to ensure that this issue is incorporated into the heart of the national curriculum for social work and health courses. The case for it is indisputable as it can only be in the best interests of employee, employer, service users, carers and society as a whole.

Mike has also developed an electronic resource made up of exercises, psychological advice and short articles designed to promote health and well-being in caring professions (contact Mike at crossbear61@ gmail.com for a copy of this resource). These resources outline strategies for individual workers on the micro level but also consider organisational management issues at the macro level in recognition of the fact that all too often the workplace can be toxic or at least anti-therapeutic. The workplace ideally needs to be an environment that values, nurtures, sustains and supports people to be the best they can so that they can give their therapeutic best to those in need of help. Sadly, in too many cases we are still a long way from the workplace becoming the therapeutic community it needs to be. This is very wasteful not only in terms of the human cost but also in terms of the financial cost arising from of staff sickness and absence. This is in the interests of no one, particularly those on the receiving end of depleted care. The last thing vulnerable people need is a burnt out and exhausted social worker, nurse, therapist or doctor. Society somehow needs to cherish rather than squander this precious spiritual energy that gets care practitioners out of bed every morning to face another challenging day where they may increasingly encounter a 'perfect storm' of ever-increasing demand but diminishing resources to deal with it.

Essentially we need a work culture that recognises that workers are human beings and that even a machine will break down if not serviced and attended to. Our societal expectation of people in caring professions, however, is that workers can give endlessly without receiving anything in return. The focus of care policy is almost exclusively on staff output, performance and conduct without any equiv-alent formal standard for the support that care professionals themselves need to receive from those who employ and manage them. Even professional bodies, for example the Health Care Professions Council (HCPC), whose purpose it is to regulate the standards relating to a wide range of care profes-sionals, has accepted in private correspondence that there is no regulatory framework for the support of care professionals nor is there any obvious intention of creating one. This surely represents a spiri-tual blindness or vacuum that can only create a vicious cycle of stress, spiritual burn-out, sickness, absence and even more depleted resources.

If care requires energy from a spiritual reserve, then unless that reserve is replenished the quality of care can only diminish and everyone will lose out. Workers are human and it is only their shared humanity that can deliver the empathy that is such a big element of care. Equally, this means that they also need an empathic work culture to avoid becoming fatigued and burnt out physically, mentally and spiritually. In the end it is impossible to keep giving spiritual energy unless you are also receiving it.

Practical Ways of Sustaining the Spiritual Energy Required for Care

We conclude by bringing together five of the more important practical applications that can be derived from an approach based on 'spiritual nutrition':

1. *The importance of supervision as emotional processing*: Supervision is often thought of as the teaching of skills or competence, whereas in fact its primary value is emotional nutrition and processing. This means that when toxic and difficult emotions are shared between supervisee and supervisor, the supervisee is able to process the emotional impact of their care work and this enables them to become mentally refreshed and spiritually re-energised so that there is a renewed capacity to carry on similar work. The risks and dangers of a lack of supervision are great. A lack of supervision can much more quickly lead to emotional and spiritual burn-out. It is helpful therefore to think of supervision as an issue of spiritual as well as of technical competence. Without a nurturing and empathic link with the mind of a supervisor, any empathic link between a care worker and those that they care for will become depleted. This means that the attitude across some care organisa-tions that regular supervision for all professionals in caring roles is a luxury rather than a necessity is in itself dangerous and self-defeating.

2. *The concept of a 'psychologically safe' working environment*: In relation to public mental health services, Seager (15) examined from a psychoanalytic and attachment theory perspective, following Winnicott (16), the factors that reduce the risk of suicide and keep all of us safe in terms of our mental and spiritual well-being. He concluded that care environments needed not just to be physically but also 'psychologically safe'. For example, he states:

> Just as the individual patient needs the containment of 'good enough' attachments to a care-giving system, so also do clinicians need the containment provided by good quality

attachments to skilled supervisors, supportive managers and meaningful policies. To be 'good enough' parents or carers, professional or otherwise, we all need the support of grandparent figures (p.272).

In the same paper Martin argues that a psychologically safe work environment requires a healthy 'professional family' where everyone feels a sense of involvement, and he continues:

The greatest risk to psychological safety for all human beings is to be forgotten, lost from view and not 'held in mind. This is arguably worse even than having a negative identity in the minds of others' (p.276).

A psychologically safe care environment is therefore one where not only the clients feel remembered and held in mind but also the staff does. One of the most practical steps therefore in ensuring good quality care is to care for the care practitioners as human beings too. However, as we have already seen, standards of care and support for care practitioners are rarely made a priority or explicitly spelled out in policies. For the sake of our collective well-being, however, it is now vital that this policy and practice deficiency in our care services culture is remedied by government, employing organisations and also professional bodies, including trade unions. In the absence of explicit standards of staff protection there will always be room for negligent and toxic work environments for our care practitioners.

3. *Looking at caseloads and workloads from a mental and spiritual perspective*: In our care services, particularly those in the public sector, the caseload allocation to any individual care practitioner is usually based upon only the physical dimensions of space, number and time: space in the diary, number of cases waiting for a service, and hours in the working day. This takes no account of the mental and spiritual energy and capacity of the practitioner. Martin (9) describes how effective care practitioners must 'tune in' with the distress of their clients and explains that this process of identification must inevitably cause vicarious distress or compassion fatigue as described by Figley (17). Martin points out that beyond the technical competence and capacity of the care practitioner as an individual, the following qualitative 'burden factors' must also be taken into account if a caseload is to be allocated in a way that is psychologically and spiritually safe:

- The emotional attachment between care-giver and care recipient
- The level and complexity of distress in the cared for person
- The reversibility and changeability of the cared-for person's problems
- The availability of other receptive minds to share the emotional burden with
- Distractions upon the care practitioner including 'top down' pressure to achieve targets
- The degree of freedom or control that the care practitioner has to escape from or get relief from the care-giving role

The more blind and emotionally illiterate we remain as a society in relation to these common-sense factors that clearly impact on mental and spiritual energy, the more likely we are to perpetuate or exacerbate toxic and neglectful public care cultures where care practitioners are overloaded and drained of the energy needed to continue healthily with the tasks that they usually are highly motivated to perform. Loading care practitioners with heavy and complex caseloads without reference to spiritual and emotional energy levels is ultimately dangerous and self-defeating for all of us.

4. *Broadening our definition of occupational health and human resources*: Traditional models of occupational health are highly medicalised and highly reactive. Usually occupational health services only get involved once a practitioner is already sick, and the aim of such services is to treat the sick individual with the aim of restoring their capacity to function at work. Our occupational health culture is therefore largely blind to the wider, systemic psychological and spiritual causes in the workplace of ill health, depletion, stress, fatigue and burn-out. This seems to be part of a wider mind-blindness in our science and in our society. However, if occupational health is to live up to its title, there has to be a paradigm shift involving an inclusion of psychological and spiritual factors alongside the biological. Even in organisations whose core business is care, to this day only lip service is paid to the psychological aspects of work environments and systems along with the morale and spiritual health of practitioners. The management practices and policy of care organisations are therefore not tied in with occupational health in a proactive way. This is a massive opportunity missed. The mental and spiritual health of workers should be the starting-point for all organisations but in particular those whose purpose is compassion and care. Occupational health, rather than operating as an isolated department taking individual referrals, should therefore be involved proactively and systemically in the design of work environments and the support of care practitioners. Such a culture of ongoing staff support would prevent health problems developing rather than reacting to them when it is too late. Occupational health could also provide a base from which to deliver ongoing staff support programmes. In the same way, Human Resources (HR) departments have a beguiling title that invites possibilities that go beyond traditional and current models. HR departments potentially could become less bureaucratic and provide some of the ongoing interpersonal back-up and spiritual support that care practitioners and their managers need.

5. *Beyond the organisation: the potential role of helplines and the internet*: The online community and the internet provide a whole new dimension in connecting care practitioners with support. We have already mentioned the on-line resources and materials developed by Mike. Organisations are increasingly using the internet and intranets to support their staff, but the problem with websites and written materials is that they can lack the interpersonal touch that is required to process live emotions fully between people. For this reason, Mike and Martin (10) also have advocated the possibility of a national helpline for public sector care practitioners, recognising that there might be an added value in terms of confidentiality in being able to seek help outside one's own organisation, especially if

that organisation is the primary source of distress. Such a helpline should be funded collectively by government, employing organisations and professional bodies. As yet, however, our attempts to stimulate the development of such a facility have fallen on stony ground.

Conclusion

Care can only be as effective as the state of mind of those providing it. To be in a healthy state to give care the human mind needs both good morale and high receptivity. These are primarily spiritual qualities that in turn depend on a constant flow of positive emotional energy, support and nutrition. If we truly want *spiritually* competent care, there is a need to include the human spirit in our models of care provision so that we can then focus more explicitly on designing ways of maintaining this flow of spiritual energy between people in care organisations. This means limiting the factors that expend emotional energy and bolstering those that supply it. This task cannot be left to the self-care of the individual practitioner alone and requires the whole organisation to provide a system of sustaining supportive relationships described by Ballatt and Campling (11) as 'intelligent kindness' and referred to by Martin (15) as the 'professional family'. In this chapter we have looked at our traditional blindness to the spiritual aspects of care provision as part of a wider scientific blindness in the West and we have suggested some practical ways of addressing this large gap in the culture of our public care services.

References

1. Seager M. Bad science and good mental health. *Therapy Today*. 2012; 23(7):12–16.
2. Capra F. *The Tao of Physics*. Berkeley, CA: Shambhala; 1975.
3. Rogers C. The necessary and sufficient conditions of therapeutic personality change. *The Journal of Counselling Psychology*. 1957; 21:95–103.
4. Rogers C. The characteristics of a helping relationship. *The Personnel and Guidance Journal*. 1958; 37(1):6–16.
5. Norcross JC (ed). *Psychotherapy Relationships That Work*. New York, NY: Oxford University Press; 2002.
6. Schore A. The effects of secure attachment relationship on right brain development affect regulation and infant mental health. *Infant Mental Health Journal*. 2001; 22:7–66.
7. Seager M. How can talking help people feel better? A review of the psychological evidence for the national Samaritans. 2010; unpublished paper available on request from the author.
8. Williams J, Mark G, Kabat-Zinn J. Mindfulness: diverse perspectives on its meaning, origins, and multiple applications at the intersection of science and dharma. *Contemporary Buddhism*. 2011; 12(1):1–18.
9. Seager M. Who cares for the carers? In Shea S, Wynyard R, Lionis C (eds). *Providing Compassionate Healthcare – Challenges in Policy and Practice*. Routledge; 2014, pp 40–53.
10. Bush M, Seager M. Why public sector workers needs a Samaritans-style helpline. The Guardian Online. 2015. Available at: https://www.theguardian.com/social-care-network/2015/jun/22/why-we-need-a-samaritans-style-helpline-for-public-sector-workers.
11. Ballatt J, Campling C. *Intelligent Kindness – Reforming the Culture of Healthcare*. RC Psych; 2011.
12. Wright, S.G. *Burnout – A Spiritual Crisis On The Way Home*. Sacred Space; 2010.
13. Menzies-Lyth I. Social systems as a defence against anxiety. *Human Relations*. 1960; 13:95–121.

14. Dobbin A. We have to be compassionate - to ourselves. *Scottish Review.* 2013; 21 May.

15. Seager M. The concept of 'psychological safety' – a psychoanalytically-informed contribution towards safe, sound & supportive mental health services. *Psychoanalytic Psychotherapy.* 2006; 20(4):266–280.

16. Winnicott DW. *The Maturational Process and The Facilitating Environment.* London: The Hogarth Press and the Institute of Psychoanalysis; 1965, p 39.

17. Figley CR (ed). *Compassion Fatigue: Coping with Secondary Post-Traumatic Stress Disorder in Those Who Treat the Traumatized.* New York: Brunner/Mazel; 1995.

Spirituality in Acute Health Care Settings

7

Janice Jones, Joanna Smith and Wilfred McSherry

Introduction

The impact of acute illness on the health and well-being of an individual can be ameliorated by drawing on individual spiritual resources. Spirituality often focuses on a search for meaning and purpose in response to changing circumstances. Spirituality can act as a resource in developing coping strategies (1). The purpose of this chapter is to outline the key principles of providing spiritual care within acute health care settings based on research evidence and using illustrations from a range of health care perspectives. We focus on understanding and meeting the spiritual needs of patients in acute health care settings. In addition, we suggest ways that staff working in acute health care settings can practice holistically to address their patients' spiritual needs. The chapter is structured around context, organisational issues, spiritual care in the acute ward (focussing on practical examples) and ethical considerations relating to addressing spirituality in acute care settings.

Context

The renewed interest in spirituality for health care and social care professionals, including medicine, nursing, social work, occupational therapy, chaplaincy and others, stems from post-modern ideas that place less emphasis on a reductionist model of scientific enquiry to provide solutions for addressing health care issues (2,3). Acute health care settings provide care across the lifespan from birth to death, embracing the full spectrum of care, including acute and critical care, midwifery, rehabilitation and end of life care. Addressing the spiritual aspects of care across such diverse contexts is challenging. There is a growing evidence base which identifies the importance of spirituality at times of illness and during life-changing events; for example, childbirth is considered a spiritually meaningful experience and occasion for both the parents and the midwife (4).

Spirituality is an important factor in patients' recovery experiences. For example, patients recovering from acute myocardial infarctions have reported the influence of spirituality on their recovery and identified spirituality as a construct that provides them with inner strength, comfort, peace, wellness, wholeness and enhanced coping (5). Spirituality can provide patients with a vehicle to experience meaning and purpose in their lives during adverse health events. These reports from patients' experiences strengthen other findings that spirituality and religion generally have a positive impact on recovery of acute health problems. Studies in the context of North American health care have further demonstrated the positive impact of personal religious and spiritual experiences on patients seeking medical care for life-changing and chronic illnesses (6,7). Traumatic experiences may elicit religious and/or spiritual expressions that reflect inner turmoil for the patient (8). Notably, the results of one detailed study, examining the associations between religion and spirituality on patients in an acute hospital setting, revealed that patients who drew on religious affiliations had shorter hospital stays (9).

Although much is written about spirituality and end of life care, in comparison there is a paucity of literature focussing specifically on spirituality in acute care settings. This is needed to support health care practice across professional groups (doctors, nurses, allied health professionals and chaplains and support workers). There is a diverse range of health care staff providing direct patient care, and each person brings their own social and professional identities and individual beliefs and values. These influence the way spirituality in care is addressed. In addition, the changing and diverse demography of the United Kingdom (UK) requires greater appreciation of individual beliefs and perspectives. For example, while the ethnicity of the UK remains predominantly white (86%), England and Wales have become more ethnically diverse with an increase in people identifying themselves as being from minority ethnic groups. In addition, 16% of the population of England and Wales are now over 65 years of age, and life expectancy has increased to 79.1 for males and 82.8 for females (10,11). Religious affiliations have decreased, with an increase in people reporting no religious orientation. Expressions of religion and faith are also increasingly diverse. There is no longer an obligation to attend church as a way of expressing faith beliefs (1). New ways of Christian worship through the emerging church movement are increasing as people make their own choices about how to engage in their religious faith (12). The national picture of demographic, cultural, religious and spiritual diversity presented in many countries today potentially impacts on the care of patients in acute health care settings.

The way patients view spirituality is highly personal and diverse. This is highlighted in the following extract that shows how a patient may experience spiritual care through everyday practice delivered with care and concern.

Illustration from practice

Researcher: Would you say that they [health care professionals] satisfactorily help you to maintain your spiritual needs?
Patient: Yes, to a large extent but they don't know they are doing it!
Researchers: So they wouldn't articulate it?
Patient: No it's through the care and concern. (15, p.236)

The practitioner driven to deliver care within increasingly demanding time constraints may still choose to approach even routine procedures from a position of valuing the individual's experience. The next extract emphasises that staff may also perceive spiritual aspects of care to be concerned with *how* procedures are carried out and care delivered.

Illustration from practice

The procedure of inserting a cannula is considered from the position of being 'done to' as a process. Alternatively, the individual's experiences and values are considered and the cannula is inserted in a manner which acknowledges the 'soul, the being of a person.' (adapted from 14, p.61)

The following section discusses the organisational issues and how they support or challenge delivering spiritual care in acute health care settings.

Organisational Issues

Health care provision within developed societies is facing unprecedented challenges including:

- An increasing number of older people accessing acute care services
- Advances in medical technology
- Changing disease profiles
- The influence of lifestyle choices on health
- Increased patient expectations
- A backdrop of a global economic crisis

This changing landscape can be challenging for health care professionals where traditional working practices must adapt and respond to change while continuing to be supported by organisational structures and frameworks. Approaching patients with respect, dignity and compassion and patient-centred care remain fundamental principles of the National Health Service (NHS) Constitution (15). Holistic, person-centred care needs to respect the patient's cultural, religious and spiritual needs. Cultural, religious and spiritual beliefs influence how individuals make sense of the world, and as dominant forces, can shape their experiences often assuming greater importance during acute or life-threatening illness. Consequently, drawing on these beliefs can provide comfort, strength and support in times of stress.

Within the UK, there has been a continuing increase in the number of patients accessing acute care services, in particular accident and emergency. Year on year admissions to acute care have risen by 60% over 5 years (16). There are a number of causes for this increase in the UK, including overall population growth, an ageing population with increasingly complex health needs, and health policies that focus on reducing inpatient care (16,17). In order to sustain the UK NHS within a limited financial envelope, 'efficiency' savings, including reducing the length of inpatient stays, have been necessary. At the same time, restrictions on social services funding have made the timely discharge of many older people from hospital increasingly difficult. Time pressure and staff shortages have presented enormous challenges to working in a person-centred way. Rushed care and task-centred practice raise concerns about opportunity to address patients' spiritual and other needs (18). Health care managers have sometimes been tasked with balancing budgets rather than placing the patient at the centre of care and service provision, as highlighted in reports of care failings in England (19,20).

Concerns about the way care is delivered to patients and the passivity of the patients' voice in care decisions have influenced the *NHS Five Year Forward View* (21). There appears to be a political, economic and ethical imperative to shift from a fragmented model of health care delivery, with separation of acute hospital, community and social care and focus on individual episodes of illness to a more integrated model underpinned by person-centred care (22). This requires a major effort from leaders and managers and requires professionals and politicians to support new models of care. In addition, for person-centred care, enshrined in the NHS Constitution (15), to become a reality, health care professionals must be given the skills, space and time to respect the dignity of individual patients and to be sensitive to, and respect, their religious, spiritual and cultural needs.

Spirituality as a construct in health care practice has been contentious in a variety of settings. Predominantly, spirituality has been criticised for the lack of an agreed definition, a position that has, according to Narayanasamy, been invented or accepted uncritically (23). In palliative care, concerns have been voiced regarding the competencies and skills required to provide spiritual care without adequate training and regulation (24). Despite these reservations, the findings of the Royal College of Nursing survey (25) indicated that nurses consider spirituality to be a fundamental aspect of their care.

The role of the nurse has been identified as supporting people who are ill and enabling people to manage health issues to achieve the best quality of life whatever their disease or disability (26). These are also common features of care provided by a number of health care professions. Acute illness can have a significant impact on a person's emotional and psychological well-being with uncertainties about recovering from the illness, and a potential impact on life and lifestyle. Patients in acute care settings are particularly vulnerable; they may be faced with a life-threatening illness, in an unfamiliar environment. Patients are often cared for in highly technological care environments, where they may also have to discuss sensitive personal issues or undergo uncomfortable and invasive procedures. In addition, patients are removed from the security of their own home and isolated from friends and family, and support systems. A shift from a predominately technically dominated and industrialised approach to a model of patient-centred care requires health professionals to have skills, time and space to elicit patients' perspectives. This includes identifying patients' concerns, exploring the impact of illness on their lives and involving them in care decisions. This approach is required in all acute health care settings, including midwifery and mental health.

Increasingly, there is greater recognition that individual characteristics such as faith, hope and compassion impact on the healing process, usually enhancing, but sometimes hindering, recovery (27). Spiritual care matters because it focuses care delivery on the individual, and recognises and utilises patients' own resources, strengths, aspirations, hopes and experiences (28). Incorporating spiritual care into practice helps health professionals to understand patients' perspectives in relation to health and illness, and has the potential to increase patient satisfaction with care delivery and increase speed of recovery.

The pressures on acute care services can be a challenge to health care professionals seeking to develop spiritually competent practice and embed holistic person-centred practice into everyday care. Spirituality is particularly relevant in health care when individuals are physically and/or mentally acutely ill or have a life-threatening condition. In these situations, the search for meaning and purpose and a framework to interpret their circumstances is particularly important (5). As well as traumatic life events, acute health care is also concerned with spiritual experiences filled with joy and hope; for example, the birth of a baby. Additionally, recovery from illness may elicit a feeling of gratitude and a spiritual response of thanksgiving. The impact of acute illness or life-threatening conditions can have a profound effect on a person's ability to cope. Resilience and coping strategies have also been acknowledged as important factors in health promotion for people with chronic diseases. Resilience, which for some can be seen as an aspect of spirituality, has been found to positively influence quality of life and health outcomes (29). Research has found a positive correlation between meeting patients' religious and spiritual needs and their satisfaction with care for significant illnesses (6). Traumatic experiences may elicit religious and/or spiritual expressions that reflect an inner turmoil for the patient (8). As mentioned, spirituality has been identified an important factor in patients' recovery experiences: a study of patients recovering from acute myocardial infarctions found spirituality as a construct provided inner strength, comfort, peace, wellness, wholeness and enhanced coping mechanisms (5). In acute mental health services, spiritual dimensions of patients' experiences have been identified as vital to recovery and the development of positive coping strategies (30,31).

Spirituality in health care practice can be understood as a way of assisting an individual to explore and find hope, meaning and purpose (1). Health care professionals are challenged with balancing policy which supports holistic person-centred practice with the reality of demands to reduce the length of stay in acute services and shortages of staff, combined with financial constraints and increased demand.

Spiritual Care in the Acute Hospital Ward

Spirituality within acute health care practice is under-researched. However, the ability to translate the constructs of spirituality to acute care is essential in order to provide compassionate, holistic care that meets the patient's physical, emotional, social and spiritual needs (2). Embedding spirituality consistently into acute care must be viewed as a continuum from admission through to discharge in order to fully support patient recovery. The provision of holistic person-centred care in an acute care environment requires health care professionals to value the uniqueness of the individual patient, treat every patient with respect and dignity and value their involvement in care (32). Acute care organisations must support a culture where health care professionals can develop spiritual competence even in the face of time constraints (32). These spiritual constructs of valuing the unique individual characteristics, connections, meaningful activities and individual beliefs provide an impetus for holistic care as opposed to a professional-dominated model of health care delivery (14). The skills suggested as necessary for spirituality to be embedded in practice include the following:

- Undertaking a spiritual history in order to establish the patient's goals and personal priorities
- Listening to the patient's fears, hopes, pain, and dreams
- Attending to all dimensions of patients and their families: body, mind and spirit
- Incorporating spiritual practices into care delivery as appropriate
- Involving chaplains and faith leaders as members of the interdisciplinary health care team (2)

The list above is dependent on the context of care and the consent of the patient, in order to avoid unnecessary intrusion. In acute settings where the priorities of care and intervention take precedence – for example traumatic injury or acute pain – the focus of care will be to address the immediate issues.

Improving the Resilience and Experience of Staff to Address Spirituality

Some people view the issue of embedding spirituality into health care practice as a problem; many don't even think about it. Additionally, health care professionals report feeling that they lack the skills and competence to address the spiritual concerns of their patients (33). The need to develop a personal understanding of spirituality in advance of developing practice skills has been acknowledged (34). The results of a survey of clinical and non-clinical staff, examining perceptions of spiritual care and abilities to meet patients' spiritual needs, found a widely held perception that delivering spiritual care was an essential component of care. However, the health care staffs were uncertain whether they were able to recognise and meet the spiritual needs of patients, suggesting the need for education and training in spiritual care (35). A contributing factor to professional burnout is suggested as being unable to treat patients with compassion and in a person-centred manner (36). Experienced and resilient health care professionals recognise the importance of delivering spiritual care and in some instances they can and do embed spirituality in their practice (1,18).

Practical workshops aimed at embedding person-centred care and the underpinning principles of compassionate care can include attention to issues of helping patients sustain meaning and purpose, essential to spiritually competent care. The *Point of Care Programme: Enabling Compassionate Care in Acute Hospital Settings* (37) was developed to improve patents' experience of care in hospital through a series of workshops for health professionals and support staff. The content of the workshops explored compassionate care and the implications of delivering this for all levels of staff, including sessions on stress and burn-out. In addition, The Royal College of Nursing has produced a pocket guide to spirituality in nursing care (38). This provides a helpful short overview of how spirituality is embedded into nursing care. In addition, an online resource, Spirituality in nursing care (50), provides in-depth explanation and reflective exercises to enhance continuing professional development. These resources can be easily adapted to the needs of other professions.

Patient and Professional Perspectives

A number of studies have explored how health care professionals can meet the spiritual needs of patients, and they provide a practical focus for discussing spirituality in acute settings (1,13,18,39). A key message within these studies is the idea that spirituality is not an adjunct to acute care, but is an integral part of the everyday ordinary encounters and interactions of an acute hospital ward. Evident in all these studies is the problem of defining spirituality, discussed in Chapter 1.

Within nursing, spiritual care has been described as 'good nursing' enacted in the everyday experience of nursing practice and embodied in the encounters where nurses listen attentively to the meanings patients place on aspects of their lives (1). Spirituality can be viewed and experienced as compassionate, whole-person care which values the individual and respects their dignity. It is expressed in nursing practice through the physical acts of nursing such as touch, helping patients to move, bathe and eat with attention to their spiritual needs (1). The following extracts illuminate how spirituality is integral to nursing practice.

Illustrations from practice

A patient was in hospital on a surgical ward, observing the busyness of the ward. He was recovering and was not worried any longer, however …

> there was one little nurse who now and then when she passed, would stop for a few seconds, squeeze his toes through the bed clothes, smile, look right at him, 'are you alright?' In that moment he knew he was the most important person in the ward for her (Adapted from 1, p.123).

A young person was receiving treatment for terminal cancer. His nurse noticed he seemed depressed and hopeless, with infrequent visits from his family. He appeared isolated.

> During a quiet moment one afternoon, she asked John if he would like her to rub his back. John readily accepted and stated that she was the first person who had touched him since he had been in the hospital. Through touch, the nurse reached out and comforted John (40, p.15).

John's need for contact had not been recognised by his family and the health care team, yet this young person was experiencing significant challenging life events.

Within occupational therapy practice, spirituality is also considered central to delivering care and therapeutic interventions. Spirituality in the context of occupational therapy is enacted through valuing the uniqueness of the individual in a person-centred, whole-person approach. An observational study of occupational therapists in acute impatient settings carrying out their daily practice identified the central role of spirituality in occupational therapy (18). The occupational therapists developed meaningful therapeutic relationships to elicit an understanding of the impact of a patient's situation. Again, spiritual constructs were embedded in the whole of care and not seen merely as 'add-ons'.

The following extracts highlight how occupational therapists embedded spirituality in an acute ward.

Illustrations from practice

How can you still manage to retain working with people's hopes, wishes and values on a busy acute ward? I don't know it just seems to be part and parcel of what we do as OTs…. With delving into their story a bit longer, or a bit deeper, I feel that's what we can extract sometimes with our initial interviews – you know getting to know the patient, spending that time, little bit more time, not great amounts of time, getting to know them and what makes them tick. And you can go back and say well did you know this? Did you realize her husband died only a month ago? Or, you know

those sorts of really important things that might have been overlooked … we do a bit more digging I feel in order to find out what really matters to the person and so we can be more hopeful.
(Interview with an occupational therapist [18, p.165]).

A common finding in all these examples from the acute care setting is that the commitment to spiritually competent practice needs to be embedded in the fabric of everyday care and central to all aspects of practice. The challenges of meeting patients' spiritual needs in the acute care setting demand attentive listening skills, to uncover what is uniquely meaningful to a patient at a time of vulnerability and uncertainty. Practicing in a compassionate and respectful manner is central to professional behaviour, as also noted by Clarke (1).

Illustration from practice

For some of the, particularly some of the trauma cases … it can be a completely unanticipated, um, catastrophic situation that's just descended on them, and, you know, particularly thinking around some of the more active people. I … a couple of cases we've had, and have at the moment where, um, mental health has been a big issue, and so there's certain elements when things are predictable but for me the important thing is that, there's not a value judgment on what has happened, it's about then kind of looking at drawing a line in the sand and saying right this is where we're at.
(Interview with an occupational therapist [18, p.155]).

In many situations, the unpredictability and uncertainty of acute care can present challenges to practice. However, as the above extract highlights, focussing on the patient's wishes and values are central to the therapeutic encounter.

There are different considerations and challenges in relation to how spirituality is addressed in different patient groups. For example, the ill child or young person presents additional challenges within an acute health care environment where staff will be working with both the child or young person and their family. Balancing the spiritual needs of both child/young person and family members is challenging. They may have different priorities and understandings of their needs and it is important to address these differences (particularly difficult at times of adolescent conflict). For the child or young person it is also important to take into consideration any developmental needs and the need to use age appropriate language and activities (41).

The role of the hospital chaplain has been identified in the context of children and young people's services; the following are examples of how spiritual care can be effectively delivered in the context of hospital chaplaincy:

- Empowering children and young people to participate in choices and decisions relating to themselves
- Creating space and using spiritual activities to promote self-reflection and contemplation, underpinned by respect
- Developing relationships with children, young people and their families which are built on rapport and trust
- Building on existing religious connections from the child or young person's faith tradition
- Using language and resources relevant to the child or young person's stage of development

- Addressing the importance of the child or young person's community in normalising spiritual care; acknowledging the novel community created during periods of hospitalisation
- Marking significant meaningful moments such a celebrating a milestone
- Acknowledging the child or young person's uniqueness and identity in the challenging context of sickness and ill health
- Using visible reminders of spiritual care; for example postcards, bracelets (39)

Research on children's spiritual care is not extensive. However, common attributes of spiritually competent care – such as dignity, respect and compassion – are shared with other age groups.

Creative activity in a safe place where connection can take place is one way to enable spiritual care for children and young people (39). The following example of the use of creativity to address the spiritual needs of children and young people could also be applied to any age group receptive to this style of intervention. For children and young people, it is important to use activities and vocabulary relevant to the child's developmental stage (41,42).

Illustration from practice

A special box, decorated by the patient and used to store special artefacts, helped a child suffering from a long-term neurological condition to address these issues. Decorating the box provided a spiritually therapeutic activity in itself, as described by the patient,

'it sparkles and makes me feel happy.'

When holding a glass pebble contained in the box,

'I'm not really a religious person, but I feel this is speaking to me'.

Exploration of spirituality and transcendence through a creative activity can be used to communicate issues of meaning and purpose in acute illness (39, p.11).

Limited research has been carried out exploring the patient's perspective on spirituality and what it means to them in terms of their health care. Various studies have explored the perceptions and expectations of health care staff, patients and the general public concerning the receipt and delivery of spiritual care. They found that, despite increased research activity in this area over the past two decades, little had changed in relation to understanding in practice. For nurses there was an understanding that spirituality was fundamental to care delivery but a limited ability to articulate what this looked like in practice. They cited lack of preparation in training and education and of guidelines to support practice (13,43,44). The principle components model for advancing spirituality within nursing and health care that was discussed in Chapter 3 provides one framework with which to apply spirituality to practice (43). The following extracts from the study provide some understanding of what spirituality means for patients and professionals.

The first example, from the patient's perspective, highlights the difficulty of expressing what spirituality is. However, the final example in this set demonstrates that a patient can recognise spirituality as part of person-centred care and know whether or not they are being attended to in a spiritually sensitive way.

Illustrations from practice

From the patient's perspective:

> I think it's personal, it depends on what the individual believes.
> (Patient [43, p.910])

> I have not a clue. I really don't know what it means. To me it's just about religion. I don't know how to describe it honestly.
> (Surgical patient [43, p.911])

> Facial, attitude, body language, her initial few sentences, gives her away. You can tell, whether she's concerned about you as individual and not as a patient.
> (Patient [43, p.912])

Second, from the professional's perspective, a range of issues was presented. The common understanding was that spirituality is personally created, concerned with meaning and purpose, and inextricably involves connection with God, or significant others or both.

Illustrations from practice

The experience of a palliative care chaplain highlights the three aspects of spirituality and spiritual care.

> The meaning purpose aspect which is most often talked about is only part of spirituality and I would say that equally at least relationships and I still struggle to find the right word a sense of transcendence awe, wonder, mystery are also important parts of spirituality and spiritual care (13, p.222).

The example suggests that spirituality and spiritual care is concerned with meaning and purpose, relationships and transcendence, however that is defined.

The above definition seems to be in stark contrast to the following one provided by a young woman who had received care on an acute medical ward:

> Spirituality I think it is personal, it depends on what the individual believes for example my mother believes spirituality to be psychic, ghosts and people coming back from the dead. Whereas I think it to be what religion you believe in your own aspects towards God.... (13, p.239)

The personal nature if spirituality is highlighted by the patient. This highlights the variable and unique nature of spirituality for the individual.

> I knew it was about finding meaning in life, whatever that might be, feeling a sense of purpose, and almost like that for me life is about finding a sense of purpose and meaning and doing what feels right what feels your life purpose or path (45, p.123).

In this last example, from a palliative care physiotherapist, the sense of meaning and purpose for an individual is linked with doing what feels right or taking the right path in life.

Spirituality and the Acute Ward Culture

So far this chapter has presented illustrative examples of how spirituality can be enacted in acute health care settings. The following section explores how spirituality is supported by organisational and management structures through leadership and role modelling. For example, neo-natal care is an ethically demanding area and a stressful environment for staff, babies and families. Spiritual leadership which nurtures a positive spirit in the workplace can provide an integrated approach to ensure the spiritual needs of all concerned are met (46). The role of a manager is essential to create and sustain a working environment that is spiritually nurturing to all concerned. Role modelling can foster the development of positive attitudes, values and behaviours which support spiritually competent care. Leaders can create a positive culture on a ward, unit or department which facilitates good spiritual care (47). However, developing such a culture depends on professional values and philosophies being put into practice. Multidisciplinary team work, which respects each team member's unique professional and personal contribution to patient care and adopts a holistic approach, provides an effective environment for good spiritual care. Ideally this care is continuous from admission to discharge (or to a peaceful death). Fragmentation of care disrupts this and can be detrimental to the patient's experience. Addressing the culture of the acute care environment, including managing transitions in care when patients have to move from one environment to another, can have a positive impact on both staff and patient experiences (18,32). Role modelling spirituality in practice by staff confident in their skills and with the resilience to cope with the challenges in acute care helps develop spiritual competence in trainees. It also avoids spirituality being seen as an optional 'add-on' to clinical practice or confined to theory (18).

Ethical Considerations for Acute Care

The context of 21st century health care, particularly in the acute hospital sector, presents many challenges to spiritually competent care in practice. Important ethical issues posed by addressing spirituality in acute health care include the following:

- Managing services with reduced resources, ensuring that care is managed effectively and efficiently
- The power relationship between vulnerable patients and health care professionals
- Skills and training of staff to avoid harm to vulnerable patients

Health care professionals are charged with managing services on limited resources. The task of managing pressures to discharge patients quickly can be in conflict with finding time and space to attend to spiritual needs. Shortage of staff can make it hard to provide person-centred, compassionate care that respects the dignity of the individual. Professional standards, values and philosophies require staff to adhere to ethical standards which specifically or implicitly include attending to spiritual needs.

In recent years, addressing spirituality and religious issues in clinical practice has given rise to a series of high profile contentious cases. These have made it more important for staff to develop competency in understanding the distinction between spirituality and religion. Professionals need to be educated to not abuse the power relationship between themselves and their patients. However, they also need not to be afraid to support people to address issues of meaning, purpose and connection in the context of acute illnesses. Integrating personal and professional beliefs and values requires health care professionals to avoid using their privileged position to promote causes not related to the health and well-being of the patients in their care. The case of the nurse who was suspended for offering to facilitate prayer for a patient heightened the concern about personal beliefs and their influence on practice (48). The potential for negative repercussions might also be linked to the recent unexpected omission of the word spiritual from the Nursing and Midwifery Council (NMC) Code (49). (As noted in Chapter 1, the General Medical Council requires doctors to include spiritual factors in their assessment of patients.)

Concerns have been raised regarding the protection of vulnerable patients from unskilled staff attempting to address their spiritual needs. Staff need the knowledge and skills and relevant training to provide basic spiritual care and to know when, with the patient's permission, to refer on to chaplaincy staff or members of the patient's faith group. This is necessary to ensure that harm is not caused to patients by staff members who are ill-equipped for the task (24). Coherent education and training strategies which are relevant to individual health care professionals' roles and responsibilities need to be developed and applied at undergraduate level and in Continuing Professional Development.

Key Messages for Embedding Spirituality in Acute Care

Addressing spirituality in acute health care settings is challenging, and a positive approach is called for in order to improve the experience for patients and staff. The key messages shown in **Table 7.1** have been explored in this chapter as positive strategies for embedding spirituality into acute hospital care.

Table 7.1 Key Messages for Embedding Spirituality into Acute Care

The patient's experience
• Patients access acute care across the lifespan from birth to death
• Patients experiencing acute ill health can experience vulnerability, needing reassurance and understanding of their unique situation and the meaning they attribute to their situation
The health care professional's experience
• Spirituality is not an adjunct to everyday practice but integral, and should be viewed as 'good' health care practice
• Skills and training of health care professionals to address patient's spiritual needs is of concern to them
• Using creativity and the everyday experiences of a patient's care to embed spirituality enhances the patient's spiritual experience
The acute ward environment and culture
• The fast pace and rushed care common in an acute hospital environment poses challenges for addressing spirituality
• The support of the organization and management in fostering a supportive culture where patient spirituality is addressed is essential
• Spirituality is the responsibility and concern of all health care workers in acute health care settings

Conclusion

This chapter has explored some of the challenges of addressing spirituality in acute health care settings and provided a positive strategy for addressing the issues health and social care professionals face. Ensuring practice is person-centred and values the patient's uniqueness is essential to embedding spiritually competent care in all settings, including acute care. Acute care poses significant challenges to health and social care teams seeking to embed spirituality in practice. A coordinated approach which values the unique contribution of each team member effectively to promote a positive environment will impact on both patients and health care professionals' experiences. Developing experienced and resilient health care professionals as champions and role models for advancing spiritual care in the acute setting is essential. Good leaders need also to influence the organisation and culture of the acute care environment. Personal and professional development of health care and social care professionals is also essential at undergraduate and postgraduate levels.

References

1. Clarke J. *Spiritual Care in Everyday Nursing Practice. A New Approach*. Basingstoke: Palgrave Macmillan; 2013.
2. Puchalski CM. The role of spirituality in health care. *Proceedings (Baylor University Medical Center)*. 2001; 14(4):352–357.
3. Ellis HK, Narayanasamy A. An investigation into the role of spirituality in nursing. *British Journal of Nursing*. 2009; 18(14):886.
4. Crowther S, Hall J. Spirituality and spiritual care in and around childbirth. *Women and Birth*. 2015; 28:173–178.
5. Walton J. Spirituality of patients recovering from an acute myocardial infarction. *Journal of Holistic Nursing*. 1999; 17(1):34–53.
6. Koenig HG. Religion, spirituality, and medicine: research findings and implications for clinical practice. *Southern Medical Journal*. 2004; 97(12):1194–1200.
7. Hill PC, Pargament KI. Advances in the conceptualization and measurement of religion and spirituality: implications for physical and mental health research. *American Psychology*. 2008; S(1):3–17
8. Ano GG, Pargament KI. Predictors of spiritual struggles: an exploratory study. *Mental Health, Religion & Culture*. 2013; 16(4):419–434.
9. Koenig HG, George LK, Titus P. Religion, spirituality, and health in medically ill hospitalized older patients. *Journal of the American Geriatrics Society*. 2004; 52(4):554–562.
10. ONS. Office for National Statistics Census 2011. 2011. Available at: www.ons.gov.uk (accessed 3/6/16).
11. ONS. National Life Tables UK, 2012–2014. 2015. Available at: www.ons.gov.uk (accessed 3/6/16).
12. Driscoll M. A pastoral perspective on the emergent church. *Criswell Theological Review*. 2006; 3/2:87–93
13. McSherry W. *The Meaning of Spirituality and Spiritual Care within Nursing and Healthcare Practice*. Wiltshire: Quay Books; 2007.
14. Nolan S. Psycho spiritual care: new concept for old content – towards a new paradigm for non-religious spiritual care. *Journal for the Study of Spirituality*. 2011; 1(1):50–64.
15. NHS England. *The Handbook to the NHS Constitution*. London: Department of Health; 2013.
16. NHS Confederation. Key facts and trends in acute care. Fact Sheet. 2015. Available at: www.nhsconfed.org/publications (accessed 29/4/16).

17. Smith P, et al. NHS Hospitals under pressure: trends in acute activity up to 2020. *Nuffield Trust*; 2014.

18. Jones JE. A qualitative study exploring how occupational therapists embed spirituality into their practice. Unpublished thesis. University of Huddersfield; 2016.

19. Francis. *Report of the Mid Staffordshire NHS Foundation Trust Public Inquiry*. London: The Stationery Office; 2013.

20. Keogh E. *Review into the quality of care and treatment provided by 14 hospital trusts in England: overview report*. NHS England; 2013.

21. NHS England. *5 Year Forward View*. 2015.

22. Naylor C, Alderwick H, Honeyman M. *Acute Hospitals and Integrated Care*. London: The Kings Fund; 2015.

23. Narayanasamy A. Recognising spiritual needs. *Spiritual Assessment in Healthcare Practice*. 2010; 37–55.

24. Cobb M. The *Dying Soul: Spiritual Care at the End of Life*. London: McGraw-Hill Education; 2001.

25. McSherry W. *RCN Spirituality Survey 2010. A Report by the Royal College of Nursing on Members' Views on Spirituality and Spiritual Care in Nursing Practice*. London: Royal College of Nursing; 2011.

26. Royal College of Nursing. *Defining Nursing*. London: Royal College of Nursing; 2014.

27. Mullan, K. Patients...not numbers, people...not statistics (2nd ed). 2009. Patients Association. Available at: http://www.patients-association.org.uk/wp-content/uploads/2014/08/Patient-Stories-2009.pdf.

28. NHS Education for Scotland. *Spiritual Care Matters. An Introductory Resource for all NHS Scotland Staff*. Edinburgh: NHS Education for Scotland; 2009.

29. Cal SF, Ribeiro de Sa L, Glustak ME, Santiago MB. Resilience in chronic diseases. A systematic review. *Cogent Psychology*. 2015; 2(1):1–9.

30. Gilbert P. *Guidelines on Spirituality For Staff in Acute Care Services*. London: National Institute of Mental Health in England; 2008.

31. Suto MJ, Smith S. Spirituality in bedlam: exploring professional conversations on acute psychiatric units. *Canadian Journal of Occupational Therapy*. 2014; 81(1):18–28.

32. Peek C, Higgins I, Milson-Hawke S, McMillan M, Harper D. Towards innovation: the development of a person-centred model of care for older people in acute care. *Contemporary Nurse*. 2007; 26(2):164–176.

33. Cockell N, McSherry W. Spiritual care in nursing: an overview of published international research. *Journal of Nursing Management*. 2012; 20(8):958–69.

34. Jones J, Topping A, Wattis J, Smith J. A concept analysis of spirituality in occupational therapy practice. *Journal for the Study of Spirituality*. 2016; 6(1):38–57.

35. Austin PD, Macleod R, Siddall PJ, McSherry W, Egan R. The ability of hospital staff to recognise and meet patients' spiritual needs: a pilot study. *Journal for the Study of Spirituality*. 2016; 6(1):20–37.

36. Lowenstein J. *The Midnight Meal and Other Essays about Doctors, Patients, and Medicine*. New Haven: Yale University Press; 2008.

37. Kings Fund. *Point of Care Programme: Enabling Compassionate Care in Acute Hospital Settings*. London: Kings Fund; 2009.

38. Royal College of Nursing. *Spirituality in Nursing Care: A Pocket Guide*. London: Royal College of Nursing; 2011.

39. Nash P, Darby K, Nash S. *Spiritual Care with Sick Children and Young People. A Handbook for Chaplains, Paediatric Health Professionals, Art Therapists and Youth Workers*. London: Jessica Kingsley; 2015.

40. Anderson B, Steen S. Spiritual care reflecting God's love to children. *Journal of Christian Nursing*. 1995; 12(2): 12–17, 47.

41. Smith J, McSherry W. Spirituality and child development: a concept analysis. *Journal of Advanced Nursing*. 2003; 45(3):307–315.

42. Hay D, Nye R. *The Spirit of the Child*. London: Jessica Kingsley; 2006.

43. McSherry W. The principle components model: a model for advancing spirituality and spiritual care within nursing and health care practice. *Journal of Clinical Nursing*. 2006; 15:905–917.

44. McSherry W, Jamieson S. The qualitative findings from an online survey investigating nurses' perceptions of spirituality and spiritual care. *Journal of Clinical Nursing*. 2013; 22:3170–3182.

45. McSherry W, Smith J. Spiritual care. In McSherry W, McSherry R, Watson R, eds. *Care in Nursing: Principles, Values and Skills*. Oxford: Oxford University Press; 2012.

46. Caldeira S, Hall J. Spiritual leadership and spiritual care in neonatology. *Journal of Nursing Management*. 2012; 20(8):1069–1075.

47. Florin J, Ehrenberg A, Ehnfors M. Patients' and nurses' perceptions of nursing problems in an acute care setting. *Journal of Advanced Nursing*. 2005; 51(2):140–149.

48. BBC News. 2009. Prayer row nurse remains defiant. Available at: http://news.bbc.co.uk/1/hi/england/somerset/7874892.stm (accessed 15/12/16).

49. NMC Code. Nursing and Midwifery Council. *The Code. Professional Standards Of Practice and Behaviour for Nurses and Midwives*. Nursing and Midwifery Council; 2015.

50. Royal College of Nursing. Spirituality in nursing care: online resource. 2011. Available at: https://www2.rcn.org.uk/_data/assets/pdf_file/0008/395864/Sprituality_online_resource_Final.pdf (accessed 14/9/16).

Spirituality and Mental Health 8

John Wattis

What Are Mental Health Problems and How Common Are They?

Physical health problems come in a variety of guises. There are acute problems like heart attacks and injuries, acute infections like pneumonia, long term infections like tuberculosis, immune problems, long-term problems like arthritis and osteoporosis, disabilities as a result of these various processes and so on. Mental health problems similarly have a great variety of presentations, causal factors and chronicity. For this reason we have avoided the use of the term *mental illness* in this chapter which, for some people, implies a simple model of causation. We have generally used common mental health problems to refer to those conditions commonly experienced to some degree by many people, especially when placed under abnormally stressful conditions. We have used the term *serious* [or *severe*] *mental health problems* to refer to generally more severe but more rare conditions. We have sometimes used the term *mental health disorders* to refer to conditions like schizophrenia and bipolar (manic-depressive) disorder (also sometimes characterised as 'psychotic' problems). We include the dementias as serious mental disorders, though they could also be classed as neurological disorders.

According to the National Institute for Health and Clinical Excellence (NICE), at any point in time around 15% of the population in the UK suffer from common mental health problems (milder forms of depression, generalised anxiety disorder and other anxiety-related problems) (1). Most of these (up to 90%) will be treated in Primary Care, often using psychological approaches of demonstrated efficacy in preference to medication. These approaches all work best if the clinician or therapist demonstrates the basic person-centred qualities of a good therapist: empathy, congruence and unconditional positive regard. The concepts of hospitality, availability and vulnerability discussed in Chapter 4 embrace these qualities. Chapter 9 also discusses the primary care context, and the growing plans for agreed care and integration of care between primary and secondary care as recommended by NICE (1).

More serious (psychotic) mental health problems affect around 4 per thousand people in a given year (2). Though this is a much lower prevalence than that for common mental health problems, the more severe problems tend to make a proportionally much higher demand on secondary care mental health services.

What's Special about Mental Health Problems?

Much of what has been written in other chapters is also relevant and important for people with common mental health problems which often co-exist with each other (e.g. anxiety and depression). They also often co-exist with physical health problems and are seen (though not always recognised or dealt with) in primary care and acute general hospital settings. Mental health problems are often associated with social prejudices which, coupled with loss of occupation in the more serious instances can result in the person feeling devalued. This is usually less of a problem for people with common mental health problems than for people with severe mental health problems, but they are by no means immune from the dehumanising effects of stigma and prejudice.

As Swinton writes in *Resurrecting the Person* (3), individuals with mental health problems struggle not only with psychological and biological factors but also with oppression, prejudice and social exclusion from 'basic sources of value' (p.10). Swinton, writing from a Christian perspective, argues that it is part of the mission of the church to offer friendship to these people. The issues around the devaluing of people can be addressed as part of spiritually competent care and are dealt with in some depth in Chapter 12 on social role valorisation. Developing the role of the church and other faith communities in supporting people with mental health issues is one of the ideas behind the Spirit in Mind project, discussed in Chapter 11.

People with mental health problems may sometimes struggle with issues of meaning and purpose and, particularly if depressed, may experience loss of hope. This means that those supporting them need to be particularly sensitive to spiritual issues, and perhaps explains why, after end-of-life care, mental health care is an area where these issues have been most researched and discussed.

An important issue to address is the relationship between phenomena that are found both in severe mental problems and in spiritual states. These include phenomena of altered consciousness (such as ecstasy), hearing voices and beliefs out of step with mainstream culture that may or may not be delusional in the technical sense of the word.

The dementias, including the commonest, Alzheimer's dementia, are another group of conditions, chiefly affecting older people, that demand a special approach to spiritual needs, not only of the people experiencing the problems directly but also of family, friends and other carers. The dementias are relatively common, affecting approximately 7% of the over 65-year-old population (4) and present particular challenges and opportunities for good quality spiritual care, based on recognition of the value of the person with dementia.

Then there is the sometimes explicit, sometimes implicit influence that religious belief and spiritual experience may have on various psychological treatments. Viktor Frankl's logotherapy (5) was based on his experiences of human suffering in Nazi concentration camps. Treatment options such as the Alcoholics Anonymous 12-step programme (6) are couched in theistic language, and various forms of therapy, e.g. Gilbert and Choden's *Mindful Compassion* (7), are associated with mindfulness, derived from Buddhist practice. Other specific forms of psychotherapy also have a religious or spiritual underpinning.

Virtually everything about spiritually competent care is relevant to working with people with mental health problems, and Chapters 11 and 12 address these issues from the perspective of mental health services. This chapter therefore focuses on three special issues: the overlap between spiritual and psychotic experiences, the issues specific to helping people with dementia and their carers, and specific forms of therapy with religious or spiritual underpinnings.

The Overlap between Spiritual and Psychotic Experiences

What psychiatrists call auditory hallucinations (hearing voices) and delusions (unshakeable beliefs, usually false and incompatible with a person's background and/or culture) are associated with a number of mental health problems. Perhaps the best known of these are the conditions labelled as schizophrenia, but some of these phenomena also occur in post-traumatic stress, severe depression, mania and other conditions.

Spiritual Experiences

People also hear voices (or a voice) as part of spiritual experience. Saint Augustine (8) recounted how he heard a child's voice chanting 'take, read' which he took to be a command from God to read the scriptures, ultimately leading to him becoming one of the most important Christian leaders of his day. The prophet Muhammad, when he was sleeping in a cave, experienced an 'overpowering embrace' and a voice commanding him 'Recite!' (9, p.21). This, to his surprise, he did, speaking the first words of the Muslim holy book, the *Qur'an*. George Fox, founder of the Quakers, reported his experience of convincement:

> then, I heard a voice which said, 'There is one, even Christ Jesus, that can speak to thy condition'; and when I heard it my heart did leap for joy (10).

Many other mystics and even the French military leader in the Hundred Years' War, Joan of Arc, have reported hearing voices or seeing visions with religious or spiritual significance.

This kind of extraordinary experience can be life-changing. Augustine became one of the greatest Christian theologians of all time, influential in the Reformation many centuries later and still regarded as one of the most important early theologians. Muhammad's experiences continued and led to the founding of Islam and its holy book the *Qur'an*. George Fox became a radical reforming preacher, pacifist and thorn in the side of the authorities, sleeping in ditches and spending years in prison. Joan of Arc was burnt at the stake as a witch when she fell into the hands of her enemies.

Psychotic Experiences

When these phenomena of visions and voices occur in the context of a psychotic state, we call them hallucinations. When strong false convictions, out of keeping with the person's background and culture arise in the same context, we call them delusional. People with psychoses often also experience their hallucinations and delusions as life-changing. Mitchell and Roberts (11, p.42) cite examples of a young man who lived in poverty, believing himself to be an 'un-empowered Messiah' waiting to be revealed at the Second Coming and another person they encountered on a psychiatric ward, a pianist who believed that an undefined 'they' had broken his fingers when he was in 'captivity'. He had been admitted to the ward via the police station but his fingers had not been broken and the problem with playing the piano seemed to be related to anxiety, distraction and being 'hopelessly out of practice'. Mitchell and Roberts point out that delusional beliefs often arise out of an attempt to find meaning in the patient's abnormal experiences. Delusions with a religious content may be built on the attempt to find personal significance in religious texts, but of course this search for meaning in sacred texts is also a normal part of spiritual experience for many people.

The 'Dark Night of The Soul'

Similar issues arise with respect to severe mood disorders and the 'dark night of the soul', originally described by the mystic St John of the Cross (12) and brought into modern perspective by Thomas Moore (13). Moore, a former monk and psychotherapist, writes a modern guide to exploring these issues. He cites examples of those who, like John of the Cross, have suffered unjust imprisonment. He mentions his namesake Thomas Moore, the 16th century theologian and statesman imprisoned and executed by Henry VIII. More recently he discusses Dietrich Bonhoeffer, imprisoned and executed by Hitler in the 1940s. He points out that in both cases these imprisonments were times of spiritual growth expressed in writings like Bonhoeffer's *Letters and Papers from Prison* (14). Others like Nelson Mandela and Terry Waite have also endured 'dark nights' of imprisonment but survived, having experienced spiritual growth through their sufferings, recounted in their autobiographies *Long Walk to Freedom* (15) and *Taken on Trust* (16).

Moore (13) discusses how life's more ordinary traumas such as unhappy marriage, divorce, bereavement, job loss and so on can also be opportunities for spiritual growth, but only by going through the 'dark night' experience, not by avoiding it. More controversially, perhaps, he suggests that depression itself (a clinical term he does not like) can be useful in this way. For the practitioner working with a person with severe depression this raises serious issues about risk. Sometimes it is necessary to contain suicide risk (as far as possible) and very often treatment with antidepressants and even, rarely, electroconvulsive therapy (ECT) may be life-saving. These measures also may enable the severely depressed person to benefit from psychological and social approaches (17, p.231). Use of medication can be enhanced by psychological and social measures and these should always be considered as part of holistic treatment.

The issue for the practitioner is where the boundaries occur (if at all) between religious and spiritual experiences.

Deciding What Is What

Based on a review of a number of sources, Peters (18) concluded that there was a continuum from normality to psychosis and that there might be little difference between the form or content of the experiences of a person with psychosis or a person undergoing spiritual experiences. The difference was in the way people responded to these phenomena. In the end it was the behaviour that followed the phenomena and how well they were integrated into the person's life that helped make the distinction.

The conundrum is well summed up by Rumi, a 13th century poet and Islamic scholar:

> The mystic dances in the sun,
> Hearing music others don't.
> 'Insanity', they say, those others.
> If so, it's a very gentle nourishing sort. (19, p.30)

What Matters in Practice

In clinical practice we are more likely to encounter those for whom the experiences of psychotic phenomena are part of a wider process, for example a bipolar disorder with phases of severe depression followed by elation, over-excitement and sometimes grandiose delusions, or perhaps someone with severe unipolar depression and delusions that they are rotting from the inside, or someone with a schizophrenia where personal disintegration characterised by disordered thinking occurs alongside phenomena like hallucinations and delusions, without any necessarily religious or spiritual content. How can we help them?

First we must recognise severe mental health problems, and where evidence-based interventions exist we must advise the person who is experiencing them and seek to engage them appropriately. This must not be limited to 'biological' interventions like medication or ECT, though these may be a necessary part of the treatment plan when people are experiencing distressing or even life-threatening phenomena. We engage the person by relating to them as a whole person, respecting their thoughts and feelings and seeking to empathise with their experiences. We also need to respect their cultural and religious beliefs as far as possible and the spiritual significance that may exist for them in what they are experiencing.

A narrative approach and narrative therapy, discussed in Chapter 4, are particularly important in this context for people with common mental health problems as well as the more severe disorders. What is the person's story from their point of view? This may be different from how we see it from our point of view. We may see their psychosis or their alcohol abuse as the main issue, they may see rejection by a spouse, loss of job or homelessness as the most important issue. That is why mental health professionals are encouraged to take a holistic view. This is typified by the process of 'formulation' taught to some psychiatric trainees. In this, the person's relevant life history and current situation including relevant psychological, social and family issues are briefly summed up, and the presenting problems are discussed together with a brief description of relevant psychological phenomena before a psychiatric *differential diagnosis* is discussed. The formulation concludes with a management plan which should be agreed upon with the person and should address all aspects of their needs, not just the diagnosis, using all appropriate means, not just medication. We would include in this traditional formulation a note of any religious or spiritual factors and the way in which their experiences are affecting their sense of meaning and purpose in life.

Sometimes agreement with people who have severe mental health problems can be impossible. Mental health professionals who judge the person to be a risk to their own health or safety or the safety of others may have to consider the use of Mental Health legislation to ensure the person is kept safe and receives needed help. This in itself can create relationship problems, though in the author's experience relationships can be rebuilt even when compulsion has been used. One of the key issues in working with any person with a mental health problem is recognising the whole person and engaging with them in a personal way with a genuine interest in how they see themselves and their problems, including any spiritual issues to do with their meaning and purpose in life. Time pressure and fragmented work patterns can make this hard to achieve, but good services should be organised to facilitate this person-to-person approach. We must regard the person as a whole person with personal resources and not just as a patient with symptoms to be cured.

Another question that people sometimes ask is whether psychotic experiences can themselves have spiritual significance. Making sense of psychotic experiences, even if retrospectively, can help on the way to recovery. This is an area where practitioners need to tread carefully, offering support as the person reconstructs their life narrative after an episode of severe mental health problem, and remembering that the story belongs to the person and not the practitioner. There are now a growing number of accounts from people who have had these experiences: see, for example, Narratives of transformation in psychosis (20).

An epilogue to the discussion on psychosis is the belief expressed by Dawkins (21) that belief in God is itself delusional. Belief in God does not meet the psychopathological definition of delusion (it is not incompatible with most people's culture or background). Andrew Sims deals with the psychiatric aspects of the question in his book *Is Faith Delusion?* (22), also concluding that religion is generally good for people's mental and physical health. A philosophical and theological rebuttal of Dawkins' views can be found in the mischievously-titled book *The Dawkins Delusion* (23).

The Special Issues Around Dementia

Dementia presents a number of special challenges. Here is a group of disorders undeniably associated with organic changes in the brain which seem to destroy the personality of the person affected. Yet, as demonstrated many years ago by Tom Kitwood and his colleagues (24,25), the suffering caused by the brain changes in dementia is made far worse by the inadequate care we offer. In *Person to Person* (24), Kitwood and Bredin stress the importance of treating the person with dementia as a person, with a family, occupational history, likes and dislikes, values, religious beliefs and so on. They make the point that as dementia advances the person becomes more dependent on others to sustain their personhood and sense of identity, yet often they end up in impoverished 'care' home situations where staff hardly know them and often have inadequate training and not enough time to get to know them. Remedies to this have been proposed and great strides have been made through staff training using methods like dementia care mapping (26) and the use of scrapbooks or 'memory boxes' to prompt both residents and staff memories. Albert Jewell has published an edited work on *Spirituality and Personhood in Ageing* (27) with a wide variety of approaches to the wider issues of ageing. There are many other works about the personal and family experience of dementia, including some from a specific spiritual or religious perspective (28,29).

Psychological Approaches in Relation to Spirituality and Religion

Several issues are explored here:

- The utility of specifically religious/spiritually-based approaches (for example the 12-step approach to alcohol problems)
- The use of therapeutic approaches that have a religious or spiritual root that has been 'secularised' (for example mindfulness-based approaches that have been developed from Buddhist tradition)
- Secular therapies that have been adapted for a particular religious group
- General or focused support from faith groups to supplement other sources of help.

Of course, things aren't really this simple but we will use these headings to facilitate discussion.

Specific Religious/Spiritually-Based Approaches

Alcoholics Anonymous and Narcotics Anonymous 12-step Approach to Alcohol Misuse or Addiction

Alcoholics anonymous provides effective help for alcoholics (30). It has its roots in the Oxford Group of Christians in the mid-1930s, and its 12-step programme contains specific references to God or 'a Power Greater than ourselves', though for many years it has emphasised that it does not require members to sub-scribe to any particular beliefs. It is worth quoting the 12 steps for anyone not familiar with them to show how religious (and spiritual) they are in tone. Their 12 'traditions' (in effect their governing document) also make specific reference to a God of love as the ultimate authority (31).

Alcoholics Anonymous 12 Steps (6)

1. We admitted we were powerless over alcohol – that our lives had become unmanageable.
2. Came to believe that a Power greater than ourselves could restore us to sanity.
3. Made a decision to turn our will and our lives over to the care of God as we understood Him.
4. Made a searching and fearless moral inventory of ourselves.
5. Admitted to God, to ourselves and to another human being the exact nature of our wrongs.

6. We're entirely ready to have God remove all these defects of character.

7. Humbly asked Him to remove our shortcomings.

8. Made a list of all persons we had harmed, and became willing to make amends to them all.

9. Made direct amends to such people wherever possible, except when to do so would injure them or others.

10. Continued to take personal inventory and when we were wrong promptly admitted it.

11. Sought through prayer and meditation to improve our conscious contact with God as we understood Him, praying only for knowledge of His will for us and the power to carry that out.

12. Having had a spiritual awakening as the result of these steps, we tried to carry this message to alcoholics and to practice these principles in all our affairs.

An interesting analysis by Rudy and Greil (32) examined the apparent contradiction between the seemingly religious nature of the 12 steps and the organisation and its insistence that it is not religious (though according to Rudy and Greil it did admit to being spiritual). They concluded that it is an *identity change organisation* which encapsulated its members and created an atmosphere of 'institutionalised awe' for the power of the group. They argued that a tension between sacred and secular was essential to its functioning and classified it as a 'quasi-religion.'

Logotherapy

As discussed in Chapter 1, Frankl asserted that meaning can be found through relationships, through a 'life's work' and even, in circumstances of great suffering, through how we respond to that suffering. Logotherapy is a form of existential therapy which involves examining our basic assumptions about life, developing insight into our beliefs, feelings and behaviour. This enables us to change and to find meaning in our lives, whatever their circumstances.

Frankl's logotherapy (5) was also consciously spiritual in its roots and concerned with the human search for meaning and purpose. In fact, Frankl believed that the primary human motivation was the search for meaning, and his approach of logotherapy focuses on helping people find the meaning in their lives.

Therapeutic Approaches with Religious or Spiritual Roots That Have Been 'Secularised'

Mindfulness-based therapies are based on the Buddhist practice of mindfulness. *Mindfulness* can be defined as the intention to observe the mind in a non-judgemental way – to step back and notice whatever arises in the mind without reacting to it. It derives from Buddhist practice as a way of dealing with the 'unsettled mind' (7, Chapter 7). The practice of mindfulness ultimately derives from the 'four noble truths' described by the Buddha (see 7, Chapter 1 for an account of these and how they relate to modern psychological understanding). Mindfulness-based therapies have been used in a wide range of conditions and are generally about as effective other psychological therapies (33). A specific form of mindfulness-based cognitive therapy (MBCT), delivered in groups, has been found to be as helpful as medication in reducing relapses in severe depression with more than three recurrences (34). The dangers of mindfulness-based therapy becoming 'fashionable' and perhaps not delivering as expected has been examined (35). A balanced view (which the Buddha would surely approve of) would be that MBCT and other mindfulness-based techniques are helpful but need to be delivered by skilled practioners and in a way that fulfils Carl Roger's core conditions (see Chapter 1).

Compassion-focused therapy is also derived from Buddhist practice, though compassion itself is a core value for many religions and social groups. Gilbert and Choden discuss the central role of compassion (7, Chapter 4) in their self-help text, which combines mindfulness as a technique with compassion (including self-compassion) as a motivation. More can be found of this approach on the Compassionate Mind Foundation website (36).

Secular Therapies That Have Been Adapted for Particular Religious Groups

Cognitive behavioural therapy (CBT) is a widely accepted and evidence-based approach to many kinds of psychological distress. The fundamental premise for CBT is that there is a reciprocal relationship between how each of us thinks, feels and behaves. If, for example, someone feels depressed, this may colour their self-evaluation ('I'm no use'), resulting in behaviour such as social withdrawal and even self-harm which can engender negative feelings and self-evaluation, perpetuating a vicious cycle. CBT accepts that it is hard to change directly how we feel. However, negative self-evaluations and other unhelpful 'automatic thoughts' can be identified and people can learn to stop these thoughts and substitute more realistic ones. This can be combined with behavioural interventions, such as learning to relax in feared situations, and with other approaches like mindfulness. CBT and its variants have become a mainstay of psychological interventions because they are relatively easy to conduct using a standardised ('manualised') approach. There are also many other variants on brief psychological interventions such as interpersonal therapy and (of course) the original non-directive therapy of Carl Rogers discussed in Chapter 1.

These approaches can be adapted to fit in with people's core religious beliefs. Harold Koenig and his colleagues have adapted standard CBT (SCBT), producing a manualised therapy, religious CBT (RCBT), which is designed to cover five major religious groupings (37) and focuses on people with major depression in the context of physical illness. An author manuscript version of this is available online (38). Initially they intended to recruit people who identified themselves as spiritual and/or religious. They had to exclude the group who considered themselves spiritual but not religious because they could not develop a manual-based treatment for this group in the same way they could for religious groups. The results of multi-centre trials of this manualised approach are beginning to be published (39,40) and first indications are that RCBT is of at least equivalent effectiveness to SCBT and that, for those with strong religious convictions, there may be merits to this tailored approach. Further results are awaited with interest at the time of writing.

As Koenig and colleagues know, spirituality is a much more difficult concept than religion to operationalise for research purposes. A spiritually competent practitioner would take into account a person's religious or spiritual sensibilities in designing and delivering therapy. In some ways, though this is hard to measure, it may be as good an approach as therapy oriented towards specific religious groupings because, as Koenig et al discuss, even groupings such as Islam, Christianity, Judaism, Buddhism and Hinduism are far from homogenous meaning that tightly manualised therapies may need modification to accommodate the individual. There may also be questions of congruence for the therapist guiding such therapy. This may be less of a problem in more homogenous cultures.

General or Focused Support from Faith Groups

Faith groups support spiritual care for people with mental problems in a variety of ways. Some provide professional counselling services to members of their own faith group and sometimes also to the wider community. United Churches Healing Ministry (UCHM, 41) in Huddersfield provides training in counselling and pastoral care. The charity also provides affordable counselling to the wider community and meets the exacting standards of the (secular) British Association for Counselling and Psychotherapy. UCHM provides training placements for students from other (secular) Colleges as well as for their own students. Though they make no secrets of their Christian foundation, they work with clients on the basis of the person's own spiritual understanding. Such services are a relative rarity (at least in the UK) but faith groups will often have people trained in counselling or pastoral care who can offer support to members.

For some people faith organisations also provide a vital source of connection, community and shared values. In the second edition of the *Handbook of Religion and Health,* Koenig et al (42, pp.300–302) report on the associations between religion/spirituality (R/S) and various measures related to mental health. For mental well-being overall, 256 of 326 (79%) studies examined showed a positive relationship between well-being and R/S. Sixty-one percent of over 400 observational studies showed that R/S was associated with lower rates of depression or faster recovery in those who were depressed. They also reported on psychosis, anxiety and a variety of other factors including a sense of meaning and purpose in life. In this last case (perhaps not surprisingly) R/S was associated with positive sense of meaning and purpose in 42 out of 45 (93%) studies examined. Their findings also cover many other areas and in some cases the findings are quite complicated. There is not space to do them justice here, but the fact that being involved in religious activity is generally good for mental (and even physical) health seems well established. It is harder to be certain about spirituality by itself because they do not distinguish between religion and spirituality, arguing that the latter is a very difficult concept to measure and that spirituality (at least for research purposes) needs to be viewed in terms of religious spirituality. A fascinating survey in the UK (43) attempted to unpick this distinction between people who adhered to a religion and people who considered themselves to be spiritual. Respondents were given a definition of religion and spirituality: 'By religion, we mean the actual practice of a faith, e.g. going to a temple, mosque, church or synagogue. Some people do not follow a religion but do have spiritual beliefs or experiences. Some people make sense of their lives without any religious or spiritual belief'. Respondents were then asked to choose whether they had a religious or spiritual understanding of life (or neither [p.69]). Over 7000 people participated in study. Thirty-five percent had a religious understanding of life and 19%

described themselves as spiritual but not religious. Forty-six percent identified themselves as neither spiritual nor religious. Religious people were similar to those who were neither religious nor spiritual with regard to the prevalence of mental health problems, except that they were less likely to have ever used drugs or be hazardous drinkers. Those who described themselves as spiritual (and not religious) were more likely than those who were neither religious nor spiritual to have ever used or be dependent on drugs and to have abnormal eating attitudes, generalised anxiety problems and a variety of other common mental health problems. They were also more likely to be taking psychotropic medication.

The authors drew the conclusion that people who had a spiritual understanding of life in the absence of a religious framework were vulnerable to mental health problems. There were a number of methodological flaws in this study, discussed in some detail in NHS News Online (44). The chief issue was that a cross-sectional study like this cannot establish the direction of causality. It is, for example, quite possible that people with common mental health problems might seek to find meaning by developing a more spiritual understanding rather than spiritual understanding rendering them vulnerable. The contrast between the findings of this study and those reported by Koenig et al (42) on the basis of a much larger volume of international (mainly North American) studies also raises the question of cultural issues and indeed whether Koenig and his colleagues are right to consider spirituality divorced from religion as a meaningless concept for research purposes.

Having cleared the academic air (or perhaps muddied the academic waters) by this consideration of the general effect that belonging to a faith organisation or considering oneself spiritual (but not religious) has on mental health, can we draw some practical conclusions?

On the whole, belonging to a religious group probably does have a positive effect on mental health. Koenig et al (42, pp.310–312), however, did find that for a minority there was a negative effect and postulated this might be related to three factors: life stress, cognitive processes and delays in seeking treatment. Overzealous adherence to religious practices might produce excessive life stress. Religion can also promote rigid thinking, legalism and disregard for individual autonomy. Some religions may have beliefs about practices that may themselves be harmful and finally some religions may discourage adherents from seeking appropriate help when they have mental health problems. On the whole, though, the part of the description in Chapter 1 of spiritually competent practice that describes supporting people connecting or reconnecting with a community where they experience a sense of well-being can be applied to connecting or reconnecting, where appropriate, with religious groupings. Of course, connecting or re-connecting with the local history society or a voluntary organisation may be equally important if that is where the person finds their sense of meaning and well-being enhanced. Swinton's *Resurrecting the Person* (3) is, in effect, a call to the Christian faith community to recognise their role in supporting people with problems, including mental health problems. Training in pastoral care, such as that offered by UCHM (41), can help ensure that people get the best possible help, though as Swinton points out (3, pp.31–52), straightforward, uncomplicated nonjudgemental friendship is one of the things that church (and other faith) communities can offer.

Summary and Conclusion

In this chapter we have examined what spiritually competent practice means for supporting people with mental health problems. Common mental health problems are mostly dealt with in primary care, often using psychological approaches. Whatever specific support, advice or therapy is used, the concepts of person-centred care and of hospitality, availability and vulnerability discussed in Chapters 4 and 9 can and probably should be applied. People with more severe mental health problems may suffer more from the dehumanising and devaluing effects of stigma and prejudice, wresting with oppression and social exclusion, issues which are dealt with, to some extent, in Chapters 11 and 12. A further issue with respect to severe mental problems is the similarity between spiritual and psychotic experiences (and, indeed, the sometimes perceived positive effects of some psychotic phenomena). This issue is discussed at some length since it important not to regard all spiritual experiences as psychotic. Dawkins' view that belief in God is 'delusional' is also addressed. Special issues surrounding the spiritually competent care of people with dementia are also touched upon.

Finally, psychological approaches to mental health problems are considered in relation to spirituality and religion. This section includes a brief look at specifically religious and spiritually based approaches to providing psychological help and secularised therapies with spiritual roots (e.g. mindfulness and compassion-focused therapy). It briefly examines religious adaptations of secular therapies and looks at the role of general or focused support from faith groups.

Because people with mental health problems are often devalued and stigmatised, they are in special need of spiritually competent care. We hope this chapter and the rest of the book will support practitioners who want to develop their competency in this area.

References

1. National institute for Health and Clinical Excellence (NICE) guidelines [CG123]. 2011. Common mental health problems: identification and pathways to care. Available at: https://www.nice.org.uk/guidance/CG123 (accessed 19/8/16).
2. Kirkbride JB, Errazuriz A, Croudace TJ, Morgan C, Jackson D, McCrone P, Murray RM, Jones PB. Systematic review of the incidence and prevalence of schizophrenia and other psychoses in England conducted for the Department of Health Policy Review Programme. 2010. Available at: http://www.psychiatry.cam.ac.uk/files/2014/05/Final-report-v1.05-Jan-12.pdf (accessed 23/8/2016).
3. Swinton J. *Resurrecting the Person*. Nashville: Abingdon Press; 2000.
4. Alzheimers Society. *Dementia UK Update*. 2nd ed. London: Alzheimers Society. 2014. Available at: https://www.alzheimers.org.uk/dementiauk (accessed 28/8/2016).
5. Frankl V. *Man's Search for Meaning*. London: Rider Books; 2004.
6. Alcoholics Anonymous (UK). Twelve-step programme. Available at: http://www.alcoholics-anonymous.org.uk/About-AA/The-12-Steps-of-AA (accessed 26/8/16).
7. Gilbert P, Choden. *Mindful Compassion*. London: Constable and Robinson; 2013.
8. *Confessions of Saint Augustine* (Xll). Available at: http://www.ccel.org/ccel/augustine/confess.ix.xii.html (accessed 23/8/2016).
9. Armstrong K. *Muhammad: Prophet for Our Time*. London: Harper Perennial; 2007.
10. Fox G. cited in *Quaker Faith and Practice* (5th ed). 19.02. (1647) London: The Religious Society of Friends (Quakers) in Britain. Available at: http://qfp.quaker.org.uk/chapter/19/ (accessed 22/8/16).
11. Mitchell S, Roberts G. Psychosis. In Cook C, Powell A, Sims A (eds). *Spirituality and Psychiatry*. London: Royal College of Psychiatrists; 2009.
12. *St John of the Cross*. Peers EA (transl). Translated from the critical edition of *P Salverio de Santa Teresa*. New York: Dover Press; 2003.

13. Moore T. *Dark Nights of the Soul*. London: Piatkus; 2004.

14. Bonhoeffer D. *Letters and Papers from Prison*. (Translated from the German; Bethge E, ed.). New York: Touchstone Books; 1997.

15. Mandela N. *Long Walk to Freedom*. London: Little, Brown and Company; 1994.

16. Waite T. *Taken on Trust*. London: Hodder and Stoughton; 1993.

17. Wattis J, Curran S. *Practical Psychiatry of Old Age* (5th edition). Oxford: Radcliffe; 2013, p 231.

18. Peters E. Are delusions on a continuum? The case of religious and delusional beliefs. In Clarke I (ed). *Psychosis and Spirituality: Exploring the New Frontier*. London: Whurr; 2001.

19. Rumi J. The mystic dances in the sun. In *Birdsong*. Barks C (transl.). Varanasi, India: Pilgrims; 2004.

20. Clarke I, Mottram K, Taylor S, Pegg H. Narratives of transformation in psychosis. In Cook CCH, Powell A, Sims A (eds). *Spirituality and Narrative in Psychiatric Practice*. London: Royal College of Psychiatrists; 2016.

21. Dawkins R. *The God Delusion*. London: Bantam; 2006.

22. Sims A. *Is Faith Delusion?* London: Continuum; 2009.

23. McGrath A, Collicutt McGrath J. *The Dawkins Delusion*. London: SPCK; 2007.

24. Kitwood T, Bredin K. *Person to Person* (2nd ed). Loughton, Essex: Gale Centre Publications; 1992.

25. Kitwood T. *Dementia Reconsidered: The Person Comes First*. Buckingham: Open University Press; 1997.

26. University of Bradford, Dementia studies. Dementia care mapping. Available at: http://www.bradford.ac.uk/health/dementia/dementia-care-mapping/ (accessed 23/8/16).

27. Jewell A (ed.) *Spirituality and Ageing*. London: Jessica Kingsley; 1999.

28. Shamy E. *More Than Body, Brain and Breath*. Red Beach-Orewa Aotearoa-New Zealand: Colcom Press; 1997.

29. Goldsmith M. *In a Strange Land ... People with Dementia and the Local Church*. Southwell, Nottinghamshire: 4M Publications; 2004.

30. Hook JN, Worthington EL Jr, Davis DE, Jennings DJ II, Gartner AL, Hook JP. Empirically supported religious and spiritual therapies. *Journal of Clinical Psychology*. 2010; 66(1):46–72.

31. Alcoholics anonymous – 12 traditions. Available at: http://www.alcoholics-anonymous.org.uk/About-AA/AA-Traditions (accessed 7/9/16).

32. Rudy DR, Greil AL. Is alcoholics anonymous a religious organisation? Meditations on marginality. *Sociological Analysis*. 1988; 50(1):41–51.

33. Khourya B, Lecomtea T, Fortina G, Massea M, Theriena P, Bouchardb V, Chapleaua M-A, Paquina K, Hofmann SG. Mindfulness-based therapy: a comprehensive meta-analysis. *Clinical Psychology Review*. 2013; 33(6):763–771.

34. Piet J, Hougaard E. The effect of mindfulness-based cognitive therapy for prevention of relapse in recurrent major depressive disorder: a systematic review and meta-analysis, *Clinical Psychology Review*. 2011; 31(6):1032–1040.

35. Farias M, Wikholm C, Mindfulness has lost its Buddhist roots and it may not be doing you good. The Conversation. 2015. Weblog. Available at: https://theconversation.com/mindfulness-has-lost-its-buddhist-roots-and-it-may-not-be-doing-you-good-42526 (accessed 25/8/2016).

36. The Compassionate Mind Foundation. Available at: http://compassionatemind.co.uk/ (accessed 25/8/2016).

37. Pearce MJ, Koenig HG, Robins CJ, Nelson B, Shaw SF, Cohen HJ, King MB. Religiously integrated cognitive behavioral therapy: a new method of treatment for major depression in patients with chronic medical illness. *Psychotherapy*. 2015; 52(1):56–66.

38. Pearce MJ, et al. Religiously integrated cognitive behavioral therapy: a new method of treatment for major depression in patients with chronic medical illness. Author manuscript version. 2015. Available at: http://www.ncbi.nlm.nih.gov/pmc/articles/PMC4457450/ (accessed 7/9/2016).

39. Koenig HG1, Pearce MJ, Nelson B, Shaw SF, Robins CJ, Daher NS, Cohen HJ, Berk LS, Bellinger DL, Pargament KI, Rosmarin DH, Vasegh S, Kristeller J, Juthani N, Nies D, King MB. Religious vs. conventional cognitive behavioral therapy for major depression in persons with chronic medical illness: a pilot randomized trial. *Journal of Nervous and Mental Disorders*. 2015; 203(4):243–251.

40. Koenig HG, Pearce MJ, Nelson B, Daher N. Effects of religious versus standard cognitive-behavioural therapy on optimisim in persons with major depression and chronic medical illness. *Depression and Anxiety*. 2015; 32(11):835–842.

41. UCHM. Available at: http://www.uchm.org/ (accessed 25/8/2016).

42. Koenig H, King D, Carson VB. *Handbook of Religion and Health* (2nd ed). Oxford: Oxford University Press; 2012.

43. King M, Marston L, McManus S, Brugha T, Meltzer H, Bebbington P. Religion, spirituality and mental health: results from a national study of English households. *The British Journal of Psychiatry*. 2013; 202(1):68–73.

44. NHS choices. Spirituality 'link' to mental illness. 2013. Available at: http://www.nhs.uk/news/2013/01January/Pages/Spirituality-link-to-mental-illness.aspx (accessed 7/9/2016).

Spirituality in the Primary Care Setting

9

Penny Keith and Melanie Rogers

This chapter introduces spirituality in primary care from the perspective of two primary care practitioners. It begins with a brief overview of some of the issues facing those working in primary care and the importance of holistic approaches to care. The current evidence concerning spirituality in primary care is then reviewed before focusing on how to operationalise spirituality in this setting. Chapter 4 provided the framework of availability and vulnerability which is particularly salient in primary care and should be reviewed by the reader as a useful framework for operationalising spirituality. A number of verbatim quotes taken from the interview transcripts from a study by Penny of ANP's in primary care have been included to offer insights into the provision of spiritual care in this setting (1).

Introduction

It is estimated that for around 90% of people their first and main point of contact with the NHS for their physical and mental health and well-being is primary care (2). Primary care includes GP practices alongside dentists, opticians and pharmacists. There are more than 8300 practices in the UK providing primary care services (3). The traditional model of primary care centres has focused on General Practice (4).

The 'Five Year Forward View' report recognised that change was needed in the health service to offer a more 'engaged relationship' to promote well-being and prevent ill-health (4). Working in partnership with local communities and a commitment to delivering care locally was seen as a priority, potentially placing primary care back in the driving seat for delivering care. To deliver the Five Year Forward View, NHS and social enterprise organisations and partnerships were invited to apply to become vanguard sites for new models of care (5). These included integrating primary and acute care systems.

Penny is working alongside colleagues in mid-Nottinghamshire on the Better Together vanguard where a new care model is being implemented. The Better Together programme brings together all health and social care organisations across the area with one aim being to focus on treatment of patients in the community (6).

Primary care needs to be responsive and flexible to meet rising demands for health and social care provision. Traditionally, patients' first contact for health needs would be to see the General Practitioner (GP). In the 1990s the role of the Practice Nurse (PN) was developed to support the GP and offer nursing care in the GP practice. With the increasing skills of nurses and the increasing demand from patients the role of the Advanced Nurse Practitioner (ANP) has developed in many areas. The patient will often present first to the GP or ANP with symptoms or concerns that are troubling them with an expectation that these will be addressed and a 'treatment' offered. The patient may then be referred to the PN for health education, chronic disease management, wound assessment, vaccinations and cervical screening, for example. PNs are often supported by Health Care Assistants (HCAs) working in primary care who are able to offer venepuncture, some health checks and new patient assessments. The primary health teams also cannot function without the full administration team, including the receptionists who have daily contact with patients and play an important role for patients. Primary health care teams continue to evolve and develop. With the Five Year Forward View there was a move to offer services which were previously provided in secondary care leading to new initiatives and services for patients provided in the community.

Most health care professionals would hope to define the care that they deliver as holistic. This, put simply, means care of the whole [Greek ὅλος] – body, mind and spirit (6). The main role of the practitioner in primary care, whether making a comprehensive assessment of the patient or offering health education and monitoring, involves direct engagement with the patient. This may include assessment of physical, social, psychological and spiritual factors and provision of appropriate support. Interactions focus on building a relationship with patients, interpersonal skills and holistic assessment of the presenting problem (7–10).

GPs, ANPs and PNs are by definition generalists and yet there is often an expectation from patients that they will also have specialist knowledge. Penny's study of ANPs has been used throughout this chapter to illustrate some of the aspects of spirituality:

> … they have this perception that because we're nurses, we can actually deal with anything that comes through the door – it doesn't matter whether it's medical or not, but oh, you're a nurse, you can deal with it! (1)

With the emphasis of provision moving from secondary care to primary care, practitioners need to develop a greater range of skills to manage increasingly complex patients (8). Primary care practitioners are expected to work in equal partnership with patients, supporting them to be self-caring where possible. This is in the face of limited resources, time pressures, and limited capacity and relatively few specialist services available at the point of consultation (11).

With the vanguard projects and the implementation of the Five Year Forward View there may be a move to federations of primary care practices and the integration of other care providers such as social care to improve efficiency and continuity.

Historically patients have only been offered 7- to 10-minute consultations with a GP. However, with the increase in health care complexity and poly-pharmacy in addition to social needs, some practices offer longer or repeat appointments for those who need them. Short consultations increase the likelihood of some aspects of care being overlooked – particularly those (like issues of meaning and purpose) requiring more in-depth discussion (11). Holistic care can be impeded by the need to focus on the presenting problem in a ten-minute consultation. This may lead to relative neglect of psychological, social, cultural and spiritual needs (12).

Clinical presentations to GPs and ANPs historically have been approached bio-medically, with further investigations, treatment or a referral often being the outcome. Many primary care presentations are multifaceted with biological, psychological, social and spiritual factors interacting with each other (13). The bio-medical model often only addresses one part of the human condition, and holistic approaches in primary care are necessary to meet patient need (13). We need to recognise the complexity of human needs and adopt a holistic approach, whichever member of the team the patient is consulting (9,10).

This means listening to patients and eliciting their concerns and anxieties in order to understand how their illness impacts on their lives. In primary care the 'ICE' mnemonic reminds practitioners of the need to elicit patients' **I**deas, **C**oncerns and **E**xpectations. It supports effective consultation and has evaluated well in studies (14). Listening to patients in this way ensures a patient-centred focus which is enhanced by shared decision-making. Listening and acknowledging patients' concerns and anxieties is also a key aspect of spirituality. One major nursing survey found that spirituality was regarded as fundamental to holistic care (15). Holistic care is partly dependent on a good long-term relationship between patient and practitioner, often involving regular engagement through intensely private and life-changing events. Holistic and compassionate care go hand in hand and help to build an effective partnership between clinician and patient (16). Working holistically needs recognition and integration of a 'body-mind-emotion-spirit' approach (17).

Towards a Bio-Psycho-Social-Spiritual Model of Care

Many presentations in primary care involve complex physical and mental health problems which may be managed with a combination of emotional support, medication, lifestyle changes (for example exercise on prescription), and psychological interventions. For mental health problems, some long-term conditions and pain management cognitive behavioural therapy, anxiety and stress management may be offered. More recently, mindfulness, which has its roots in Buddhism, has been successfully adapted into secular health and social care. The importance not just of physical care but mental well-being is becoming more familiar within primary health care and connects to spirituality (18). Some health care providers have opened recovery colleges focusing on well-being where patients can self-refer (19,20). These colleges often offer social support to reduce isolation, stress and low mood and help to increase self-confidence, self-esteem and resilience. There is often a focus on spirituality through an ethos of inspiring hope, meaning and purpose (19,20). Health and social care providers must go beyond dealing only with physical or mental health issues. They should 'enable people to live their lives as they wish, to work towards their goals and to have valued and rewarding relationships' (19, p.8). This can be achieved by supporting people to manage their symptoms and keep themselves well and giving opportunities to retain or (re)gain a meaningful life (see Chapter 12 on social role valorisation). In addition to this, there needs to be a commitment to support staff to stay well and to be resilient, alongside carers, families and friends of people who use services (see Chapter 6). Recovery or well-being plans encourage people to identify and focus on their goals, aspirations and dreams. A number of modules are offered through the recovery colleges. In the Nottinghamshire Recovery College this includes a module which delivers an introduction to spirituality and religion in health care, and also mindfulness workshops (19,20).

Spirituality in Primary Care – Evidence Base

There is a great opportunity to deliver spiritual care alongside meeting people's physical and mental health care needs in primary care. Baird et al (21) recognised that the primary care workload has increased in both volume and complexity, however this has not been matched by a commensurate increase in funding or staff. The Five Year Forward View report suggested the new models of practice referred to earlier in this chapter (4). These models require secondary and primary care providers to work more closely together enabling groups of GPs to combine with nurses, other community health services, hospital specialists, mental health and social care to create integrated out-of-hospital care. The growing recognition of the value of social prescribing may give additional support. Social prescribing was proposed by the Department of Health in the form of social prescriptions for people with long-term conditions. This was then developed to link patients in primary care with support in their local community. Alongside existing treatments and medication, social prescribing is a non-medical referral option for primary care professionals to help patients improve their health and well-being.

Many practitioners within primary care acknowledge a lack of education and knowledge around delivering spiritual care. Penny and Melanie have both undertaken research in the UK around spirituality in primary care with ANPs and ANP students (1,22). Both studies investigated the lived experience of the practitioners in relation to their spirituality. Participants in both studies were keen to integrate spirituality into their practice. However, some felt that they lacked sufficient understanding of their own spirituality and the spiritual needs of patients to be able to offer this care. Participants in both studies were able to offer examples of spiritual care within a primary care consultation despite having received minimal formal spiritual education or preparation during their general nurse training.

Participants in both studies recognised the need to identify spiritual needs in patients as well as recognising their own spiritual needs. Practitioners saw themselves as being on a continuing personal journey which was reflected in their practice:

> I think as you get older, you sort of understand things a bit better, you reflect on things in the past and you realise that perhaps you didn't behave the way you should have done, and given the scenario again, then you would probably change your actions. So I think it's probably a constant life-changing thing from now on, forward, as well (1).

Melanie's study offered a conceptual understanding of spirituality, suggesting it was influenced by context and emotional involvement (22). The framework of availability and vulnerability presented in Chapter 4 offers a conceptual framework for practitioners to operationalise spirituality in practice.

Penny and Melanie both found that participants were keen not to conflate spirituality and religion and were able to offer definitions recognising the individuality and uniqueness of spirituality and its relationship to hope, meaning and purpose (22). Interestingly, religious background was not a major factor in the participants' spiritual journey or their self-perceived ability to offer spiritual care to their patients (1). This was an important finding, as sometimes practitioners view spiritual need as being synonymous with religious need. Those who are not themselves religious then do not feel this is something that they can offer. However, our respondents felt differently, as typified by this statement from a practitioner:

> Well, if they're there, talking to you, they're asking for you, your help, not someone else's. I'm sure most people are quite capable of deciding, I need to speak to a priest! But if they're sitting there talking to a nurse, they're not saying, I need to see a priest; they're saying, I want to talk to you about this. Then you're there, so it's your role whether you want to do it or not really (1).

Additional challenges to providing spiritually competent care are reported to be lack of education, lack of appropriately trained staff, time and resources (7,9,23,24). In a time of cost improvement, where the focus is on delivering more for less, it is often difficult to offer care that is not a reaction to the immediate presented problem. The caricature of the practitioner writing a prescription before the patient has sat down is not so far from the reality. In an ethos of targets and numbers it is difficult to take time to explore wider than the presenting symptom(s). However, most would acknowledge that time taken in the early stages of a consultation to provide holistic care does reap benefits and saves repeat attendances and ongoing problems; it also increases patient satisfaction. The environment can also be a barrier to delivering holistic care. Most primary care settings do not encourage opportunity for conversations and the development of relationships. Patients see themselves as passive recipients of treatment. They are not encouraged to recognise that there may be a spiritual element to their concerns. These spiritual concerns about meaning and purpose emerge, often quite dramatically, in times of illness or crisis. In secondary care spiritual care is often supplemented by specialist chaplaincy teams, but in primary care this is less common.

Spirituality and Education

A barrier to integrating spirituality in practice that is often cited is the lack of formal education (7,25,26). The Royal College of Nursing carried out a survey of 4000 nurses which found that 80% of those surveyed felt that spirituality should be taught in nurse education as it was part of the core practice of nursing (27). Both Penny and Melanie found that the ANPs they interviewed were willing to meet patients' spiritual needs even though they did not feel that they had been adequately prepared (1,22).

> I think with nursing care that people can access us when they're in crisis; I mean, you know, they can come in and say, 'Oh, I need to see someone. I need to see someone today!' and often you are dealing with someone who's having some emotional spiritual crisis and I don't have any resources to help them (1).

Both Melanie and Penny have taught sessions on spirituality for students on nurse practitioner courses. These always evaluated well and often students fed back that this was the first time they had been given the opportunity to reflect on their own spiritual thoughts and beliefs. They often reflected that they had been confused about what spirituality was and how to integrate this into their practice. After the teaching they felt much more comfortable with the concept and acknowledged that they often had been providing spiritually competent care without realising it. Understanding what spirituality is and one's own thoughts around spirituality is a first step to practitioners being able to deliver spiritually competent care. Teaching on spirituality should be seen as an essential element of health care curricula:

> The specific session that we did with you, everybody absolutely loved it, everybody's really enjoyed that. It was one of those things that I think it would be fair to say of most people, it's not something you actually give much head space to. So to have an intense session of it, where that was what the whole session was about, was really good and was memorable (1).

In America, medical education has recognised that spirituality is an integral part of holistic care, with 100 out of 150 medical schools in the USA reporting that they now include spirituality in their programmes and of those 100, 75 make taking at least one module on spirituality compulsory (28).

Spiritual Competence

Several competency documents support the integration of spirituality into practice (29,30). These include a suggestion that clinicians should recognise patients' rights to express their spiritual beliefs, assist patients and their families to meet their spiritual needs, assess the influence of patients' spirituality on their health care behaviours, and incorporate spiritual needs and beliefs if appropriate into care plans (29,30).

Although GPs generally agreed that they should support their patients' spiritual well-being, they reported that they lacked the knowledge and skills to deliver this care (31). Many studies confirm this lack of knowledge as a significant contributory factor in why GPs and ANPs do not deliver spiritual care (23,28,31–33). However, the studies also raise other concerns and issues which contribute to health care practitioners avoiding spiritual care needs. Monroe et al reported that 84.5% of their respondents believed spiritual care was important in practice yet only a third actually provided this (28). It seems unlikely that this dissonance between what practitioners believe and what they practice is purely related to educational preparation, given the other findings of the studies about personal discomfort or spirituality being a private matter for patients.

Self-awareness and self-understanding are important to the individual. If there is a personal examination of our own beliefs and values, we may then be better able to understand others. By recognising our own biases and prejudices we

> … ensure that we do not impose our own values and beliefs … Self-awareness should enable the nurse to adopt a non-judgmental approach (6, p.31).

Primary care offers opportunities to provide spiritually competent care. Practitioners need to recognise the importance of offering compassion and how this is integral to spiritually competent care. *Compassion in Practice* (34) proposed the 6 C's (care, compassion, competence, communication, courage and commitment) should be integrated into practice as a way of delivering compassionate care. Spirituality was not openly acknowledged in the strategy but it could be argued that it is difficult to exclude spirituality from compassionate care (24). *Spiritual Care Matters: An Introductory Resource for all NHS Scotland Staff* (24) is based on the premise that health requires a spiritual and compassionate element alongside the physical, psychological and social elements in order to describe a holistic or whole-person approach to health and health care. To deliver this care all health care practitioners need to be spiritually competent:

> Those privileged and entrusted to provide care in the NHS must further develop and sustain their capacities to offer with equal seriousness, the appropriate spiritual and religious care (24, p.20).

Meeting patients' spiritual needs has a positive effect on their physical and psychological well-being. Koenig writes that there is quantitative and qualitative evidence that, what he describes as, 'religion/ spirituality' has a positive impact on well-being and helping individuals to deal with internal and external adversities (35).

Intelligent Kindness

The culture of health care was brought to the fore by the Francis report (36). This report highlighted the negative culture of poor care and a lack of compassion that was evident in many of the health care professionals working in the Mid-Staffordshire Trust. Ballat and Campling stated the case for examining whether the culture within the NHS was promoting kindness or cruelty (37,38). Part of the response to the Francis report was to introduce more regulation and metrics whilst at the same time seeking to find financial efficiency savings. The risk was that this would compound the problems. Ballat and Campling argued for the need to create a culture of *Intelligent Kindness* to 'nourish compassionate health care' (37, p.179). Their challenge was to move away from the blame culture that focused on poor practice and rigid control to supporting and enabling staff to deliver compassionate care. They argued that most people respond to kindness and that if individuals felt safe and cared for they would be able to be kind and compassionate themselves. Health care professionals needed to reinstate 'attentive kindness' (37, p.37) as a main cultural driver in delivering their duty of care. By placing kindness back at the centre of care a 'virtuous circle' (37, p.43) would be set in motion. This virtuous circle could then improve staff morale, lower stress and improve sickness rates. The initial kindness would lead to attentiveness, which would then enable attunement and build trust, generating a therapeutic alliance and improving outcomes. This would reduce anxiety and defensive practice, reinforcing the conditions for kindness and completing the virtuous circle. There was no overt mention of spirituality but what was advocated can aptly be described as a spirit of kindness.

Availability and Vulnerability

Melanie's framework for providing spirituality competent practice, based on availability and vulnerability, has transferability for all primary care practitioners. The framework, explored in depth in Chapter 4, suggests that to be welcoming, to offer attentive listening, prescencing, empathy and compassion are all fundamental aspects of spiritually competent practice (22).

The consultation is where patients can be listened to and understood by the health care professionals' welcome, acceptance and prescencing. The way the consultation begins and how the patient is welcomed often influences the whole consultation. By consciously welcoming each patient and by being open and willing to be available to patients and to truly listen, the ground is laid for a mutual exchange based on equality and acceptance.

Key to welcoming a patient is to truly listen. Attentive listening means really hearing what they are saying rather than simply listening to the words. It is this conscious listening, caring and prescencing that can meet a patient's spiritual needs (24).

Melanie's theme of professional vulnerability is demonstrated through empathy. By showing empathy the practitioner also shows human connection (22).

Human-to-Human Connection

Belonging and connectedness can be seen as basic human needs. Maslow's Hierarchy of Needs includes 'belongingness' (cited in 39, p.130). This need to belong was noted by Bowlby, who developed attachment theory (cited in 40, p.486). Attachment behaviour, originally discussed as a feature of child development, is manifested throughout a person's life. Once a person's physiological and safety needs are secure there is a need for belonging and love. People need to feel needed and accepted by others (39). Part of truly compassionate care is demonstrating unconditional altruistic love. It is through a therapeutic relationship that the patient and health care professional make this connection which in itself can be seen as a spiritual phenomenon.

Melanie's framework of availability and vulnerability addresses issues of emotional connectedness (22). Practitioners have to connect on a human level to reach out to another person and be able to understand their spiritual care needs. This will then support the patient to find hope, meaning and purpose. A respondent in Penny's study described this connectedness as

> ... underneath, there's ... almost an electricity between you; there's a bonding between you and your patients. And occasionally it doesn't come off, occasionally you get a person that you find it very difficult to bond with, but there's still an emotional interaction ... It becomes more difficult, but 90% of the time, let's face it, it's a rewarding interaction. I suppose that feeds back on your own self esteem at the end of the day. Maybe that's what it's all about. I want to be loved! (1)

However, this can be at a cost and so many practitioners are aware that they put in boundaries. These are overt in professional codes of conduct but also in both Penny and Melanie's studies the ANPs acknowledged that they used their own boundaries to protect themselves against burnout (1,22).

> I've done that under pressure, thinking, if I say this, the patient's going to fall to bits! So ... and I just can't do it today, either because I recognise I wasn't in the position to give out more at that point, or

practically I wasn't. And, you know, you can do it dead easily in consultations and just sort of think, right, and so let's do your blood pressure next and just get onto the next thing, and the patient closes down (1).

In delivering holistic care there is a significant risk of burnout (see Chapter 6). It is common within health care (24,41). Wright describes burnout as a 'spiritual crisis' which impacts the professional's meaning and purpose and leads to the struggle to work (41). It is a fine balance between being available and giving of self and becoming drained and unable to cope. Giving too much of self or being constantly available and present to patients could become draining and unsustainable. For many clinicians there is a desire to be with the patient, particularly when delivering end-of-life care (42). Delivering compassionate care can be costly:

> … one of my GP colleagues who was famously very good with all people with mental health problems and just got burned out on it, you know, and ended up being very ill. And it makes me very wary, you know, that I don't want to deal with it (1).

This may also be because health care practitioners see themselves as the givers and may not be so good at looking after themselves:

> When it comes to asking for emotional support, I think generally we're very bad at that, because we see ourselves as actually giving it and not receiving it. And then it's kind of a sort of a weakness, isn't it? … And I think that's a failing with nurses, and it's a failing with me personally, you know, I'll sort of keep going until I cave in, because, you know, you just don't ask for help, do you? Because you're expected to give it not receive it (1).

However, it can be so rewarding if the practitioner is able to keep that balance between being available and vulnerable:

> I think that's where, as nurses, we're privileged, because we're used to listening to people and gradually that, for most but again not all nurses, I suspect, but for most nurses I think our comfort zone's moved into a different place, so people being upset and people, you know, getting to us and feeling a bit of an emotional thing going on, it's not as scary as it was before we were nurses (1).

Melanie's framework describes availability as

- To be available to ourselves in our inner lives continuing … to be self-reflective and self-accepting, embracing spirituality (broadly defined as understanding of one's meaning, purpose and direction in life) as key to our inner journey.
- To be welcoming to patients, offering time, acceptance and understanding.
- To offer care and concern for patients through active participation, creating a safe place for patients to tell their story as it is.
- To be available to develop … practice in response to the needs of the community and patients (22).

And the framework describes vulnerability as

- To be teachable; accepting the vulnerability of the (health care professional) role and the reality that within their work they will never 'know all'.
- To be willing to embrace accountability: engaging in supervision, reflection and admission of mistakes and being receptive to constructive criticism.
- To be willing to be an advocate for patients. If necessary questioning authority, being honest and truthful with the best interests of the patient at heart.
- To be vulnerable and authentic in the approach to care of patients.
- To be willing to be challenged and questioned without defensiveness (22).

For the health care professional to offer care which encompasses spirituality these elements may be one way of doing this.

Understanding that spirituality is not about religion but about hope, meaning and purpose, understanding of loss and suffering, one's own mortality and sources of hope is an important step to being able to deliver spiritually competent care. Once this is recognised and understood by the health care professional, spirituality becomes more accessible and something that they would have some empathy with

> … made me think more about the fact that spirituality isn't just about religion, but it's about what … yeah, the way you think and the way you process things with relation to how you feel in your life and more of the meaning of it all (1).

For some this may be framed in a faith and in the context of organised religion. Others will have their own belief system as the basis for their understandings of meaning and purpose. Again, once this has been acknowledged, the health care professional can understand what spiritual care can offer:

> I would want somebody with an emotional dimension, with a spiritual dimension, to be dealing with the people I love. I wouldn't want them to be dealt with by somebody who, you know, wipes their bum and can deal with their cardiac monitor; there's something missing from them (1).

Alongside burnout are the issues of time constraints for all health care practitioners and especially for those working to set consultation times in general practice. Melanie found this within her own study and this was also confirmed by Vermandere's review (22,31). Alongside the appointment times are the external pressure of metrics which deliver rewards and incentives such as the Quality outcome Frameworks (QoFs, outlined in the General Medical Services contract). The focus of such incentives is to deliver quality care but by focusing on particular aspects of care, they can lead to others, including meeting spiritual needs, being neglected.

A number of authors suggest practitioners are personally uncomfortable dealing with spirituality, which they believe should be a private issue (23,28). This might limit spirituality being addressed and spiritual needs being met. This may lead to practitioners waiting for the patient to make a specific request (31).

However, Tanyi et al found that simply 'being present' with the patient could be a very powerful spiritual intervention (43). Sometimes this reluctance to raise spiritual issues may be the result of the clinician's own fear (28,23,33).

Wynne suggested that, whereas nurses always traditionally delivered holistic care, with increasing emphasis on technology and science there had been a move to nurses and particularly ANPs becoming much more aligned to the traditional bio-medical model (22,42,44). Vermandere et al suggested that a bio-psycho-social-spiritual model was more truly holistic (13,31).

Ellis et al (33) cited cultural sensitivity as a potential barrier to offering spiritual care Almost all of the GP studies reviewed by Vermandere et al (31) mentioned different belief systems as a barrier to spiritual discussion. Many clinicians work with a diverse population of patients and need to be able to accommodate a variety of spiritual and cultural beliefs:

> I think because you see such a wide diversity of patients you're probably more likely to be involved in people's different belief systems than you were if you say, for example, worked in [well-known national supermarket]; you're not going to get that same exposure (1).

This means that practitioners have to be flexible with regard to cultural and spiritual issues and to take a lead from the patient when they are unsure in these areas.

To deliver truly holistic care, spiritual needs should be assessed. There are tools that have been developed for spiritual assessment ('FICA' and 'HOPE' tools cited in 22). However, clinicians have reported that these can be cumbersome to use in practice and seem false (31). Some of the studies in Vermandere's review highlighted that GPs often felt uncomfortable initiating a discussion about spirituality and preferred this to be patient led (31). This was because they were afraid of causing unnecessary distress to the patient or of seeming inappropriate or being misinterpreted. Melanie has suggested that this can be better done through presencing (22). Presencing or 'being there' with the patient can be central to health care professionals operationalising spirituality (43).

In times of crisis or extreme emotional distress patients may ask 'Why is this happening?' and questions such as this can then provide cues for discussing spirituality (23,31,33,42,43). Stranahan argued that those who have their own personal spirituality are more able to pick up on these cues, and Vermandere found that GPs who were more spiritually inclined were more likely to address patients' spiritual needs (31,32). However, most are aware of the boundaries imposed by their professional codes of conduct:

> Make sure that you do not express your personal beliefs (including political, religious or moral beliefs) to people in an inappropriate way (45, p.15).
>
> You must not express your personal beliefs (including political, religious and moral beliefs) to patients in ways that exploit their vulnerability or are likely to cause them distress (46, p.1).

This can add to clinicians shying away from discussing spiritual concerns for fear of not adhering to their codes (31).

Patient Expectations

Patients are actively encouraged to be partners in health care with the call for – 'No decision about me without me' to be paramount (4,47). This puts increasing demands on health care professionals to meet their rising expectations. Ellis and Campbell found that patients thought that their GPs would not want to discuss their spiritual needs and indeed could even be hostile not because they would not want to discuss such matters but because they did not have the time (33). Patients were also reluctant to show their vulnerability by introducing spirituality into their consultations. In response to this, Ellis and Campbell advised developing the therapeutic relationship over time to let this discussion happen more naturally, otherwise if neither GPs nor patients wanted to initiate them, these conversations would never happen (31,33).

Spiritual care is fundamental to holistic practice. It appears to include the core skills of nursing, for example compassion, prescencing, individual care, listening and respect. It is integral to the way health care professionals interact with patients. It requires a level of maturity and recognition of the importance of spirituality to patients. By using listening, prescencing, empathy, compassion, humanity and care (26) practitioners can offer meaningful and individualised spiritual care to their patients. When this is given patients often recognise this spiritual care for themselves.

Chaplaincy in Primary Care

There has not been a national acknowledgement that spiritual care is central to primary health care in the same way that it is central to end of life care (42,43) and to a lesser extent in mental health care (35,48). However, there are areas that are developing within discrete communities. The Professional Association of Community Healthcare Chaplains (PACHC) aims to facilitate whole-person care in primary health care and to support GPs and their colleagues to deliver this (25). The PACHC acknowledges that the providers of primary care are the first point of contact for physical and mental health and well-being concerns for most non-urgent cases (25). Health care professionals within GP practices aim to resolve problems locally, including through services provided by the practice. Community-based care is increasingly the preferred means of providing care for the majority of longer term and mild to moderate conditions. This enables people to keep their normal routine, staying close to family and friends (4,49).

Some primary care practitioners have employed their own chaplains (25). The community chaplaincy national programme has implemented the health care chaplaincy training and development unit of NHS education for Scotland (24) to standardise the training for chaplains employed in primary care. This is supported by the Scottish government and is based on a philosophy of hope – that the person begins to find meaning, control and confidence in themselves and hope (24).

The PACHC (25) found that that community health care practitioners did want to deliver this whole person care but there were barriers to prevent this happening – difficulty understanding the concepts of spiritual care, not being familiar with the vocabulary of spirituality, feeling safe with providing a biomedical service and being concerned that to offer this spiritual element would increase the time needed to spend with patients.

Conclusion

In many ways primary health care has not kept up with recent thinking. There is a rapidly growing body of literature and evidence about the need for spiritual care. It supports other aspects of patient care and brings about better outcomes, and this is often now seen as integral to good quality care (7,24-26,43). Stobart suggests that

> … spiritual care is like describing the shape of water. Water takes the shape of the vessel that contains it. I believe that spiritual care is at the heart of everything that happens in health care (24, p.4).

In order for this to occur practitioners need to understand what spiritually competent care is and be prepared to deliver this in a way that is meaningful. This will mean working in partnerships with charities, voluntary organisations and spiritual care providers and across traditional boundaries with primary and secondary care (4). Practitioners will need to work in a more integrated way to offer physical, mental and social health care. Services will need to be integrated around the patient and this will offer enormous opportunities for primary care to offer authentic holistic care. Building on the spiritual care models used in end-of-life care spiritual care could become commonplace in primary care. Primary care itself will move from the traditional GP-led model to a leadership model which includes nurses, therapists and other community-based professionals (4). By introducing new roles and acknowledging the skills needed to deliver health care in the 21st century, primary care could encompass the bio-psycho-spiritual model. Melanie's framework as described further in Chapter 4 is an accessible and helpful way to deliver spiritual care (22). In this way practitioners can be supported to offer authentic holistic care and see the benefits of this for both their patients and themselves:

> I suppose it [spirituality] ties in with why I wanted to be a nurse … I think in some people there is an inherent need to give this love, this compassion, that there's an overflow; there's this, come on – come and get it! … It's a respect, it's a love, it's a desire to help, but I don't know where it comes from. But, if you subscribe to it, you become a nurse, in effect. You know, it's like a club (1).

References

1. Keith P. A phenomenological enquiry into the lived experience of nurse practitioner students in relation to their spirituality. Unpublished Masters' Dissertation. London: Southbank University; 2007.
2. Health and Social Care information Centre. Primary care. Available at: http://www.hscic.gov.uk/primary-care (accessed 16/6/16).
3. Department of Health. Guide to the healthcare system in England. 2013. Available at: https://www.gov.uk/government/uploads/system/uploads/attachment_data/file/194002/9421-2900878-TSO-NHS_Guide_to_Healthcare_WEB.PDF (accessed 16/6/16).
4. NHS England. Five year forward. Corporate Report CQC, Monitor, NICE, PHE, NHS England, NHS TDA, HEE. 2014. Available at: https://www.england.nhs.uk/wp-content/uploads/2014/10/5yfv-web.pdf (30/6/16).

5. NHS England. New care models – vanguard sites. 2015. Available at: https://www.england.nhs.uk/ourwork/futurenhs/new-care-models/ (accessed 16/6/16).

6. Better Together Programme. Better together in Mid-Nottinghamshire. 2016. Available at: http://www.bettertogethermidnotts.org.uk/ (accessed 16/6/16).

7. Narayanasamy B. *Spiritual Care: A Practical Guide for Nurses.* Lancaster: Quay Publishing and Nottingham BKT Information Services; 1991.

8. Goodwin, N. Curry, N. Naylor, C. Ross, S. Duldig, W. Managing People with Long Term Conditions. 2011. London: King's Fund. Available at: http://www.kingsfund.org.uk/sites/files/kf/field/field_document/managing-people-long-term-conditions-gp-inquiry-research-paper-mar11.pdf (accessed 16/6/16).

9. Murray S, Kendall M, Boyd K, Worth A, Benton T. General practitioners and their possible role in providing spiritual care: a qualitative study. *British Journal of General Practice.* 2003; 957–959.

10. Barr A, Stainsby K, Dryden S, Aston J. *General Practice Advanced Nurse Practitioner Competencies.* London: Royal College of General Practitioners; 2015.

11. Madan A. *General Practice View.* London: NHS England; 2016.

12. Shuler P, Davis J. The Shuler nurse practitioner practice model: a theoretical model for nurse practitioner clinicians, educators and researchers. *Journal of the American Academy of Nurse Practitioners.* 1993; (5):1–18.

13. Ogden J. *Health Psychology – A Textbook.* Maidenhead: Open University Press; 2007.

14. Mattys J, Elwy E, Deveugele M. Patients' ideas, concerns and expectations (ICE) in general practice - impact on prescribing. *British Journal of General Practice.* 2009; 59(558):29–36.

15. McSherry W, Jamieson S. An online survey of nurses' perceptions of spirituality and spiritual care. *Journal of Clinical Nursing.* 2011; 20(11):1757–1767.

16. World Health Organisation. *People Centred Health Care: A Policy Framework.* Geneva: WHO; 2007.

17. Montgomery-Dossey B, Keegan L. *Holistic Nursing - A Handbook for Practice.* (6th edition). Burlington: Jones and Bartlett Learning; 2003.

18. Department of Health. *No Health Without Mental Health: Delivering Better Mental Health Outcomes for People of all Ages.* London: Department of Health; 2011.

19. Nottinghamshire Healthcare NHS Foundation Trust. Nottingham Primary Health Wellbeing and Recovery College. Nottingham: NHFT. 2015a. Available from: http://www.nottinghamshirehealthcare.nhs.uk/our-courses-primary-recovery (accessed 17/6/16).

20. Nottinghamshire Healthcare NHS Foundation Trust. Recovery Prospectus. Nottingham: NHFT. 2015b. Available from: http://www.nottinghamshirehealthcare.nhs.uk/learning-and-development (accessed 17/6/16).

21. Baird M, Blount A, Brungardt S, et al. Joint principles: integrating behavioral health care into the patient-centred medical home. *The Annals of Family Medicine.* 2014;1;12 (2):183–185.

22. Rogers M. Spiritual dimensions of advanced nurse practitioner consultations in primary care through the lens of availability and vulnerability. A hermeneutic enquiry. Doctoral thesis. 2015. Available at: http://eprints.hud.ac.uk/28469/.

23. Ellis M, Campbell J, Detwiller-Breidenbach A, Hubbard D. What do family physicians think about spirituality in clinical practice? *The Journal of Family Practice.* 2002; 51(3):249–254.

24. NHS Scotland. *Spiritual Care Matters: An Introductory Resource for all NHS Scotland Staff.* Edinburgh: NHS Education for Scotland; 2009.

25. Professional Association of Community Healthcare Chaplaincy. The case for community healthcare chaplaincy: facilitating whole-person care in general practice. PACHC. 2012. Available at: http://www.pachc.info/ (accessed 23/6/16).

26. Harrison J. Spirituality and nursing practice. *Journal of Clinical Nursing.* 1993; 2:211–217.

27. McSherry W, Jamieson S. The qualitative findings from an online survey investigating nurses' perceptions of spirituality and spiritual care. *Journal of Clinical Nursing*. 2013; (21–22);3170–3182.

28. Monroe M, Bynum D, Susi B, et al. Primary care physician preference regarding spiritual behaviour in medical practice. *Archives of Internal Medicine*. 2008; 163:2751–2756.

29. Royal College of Nursing. *Spirituality in Nursing Care: A Pocket Guide*. London: Royal College of Nursing; 2011.

30. Royal College of Nursing. *Nurse Practitioners – an RCN Guide to the Nurse Practitioner Role, Competencies and Programme Accreditation*. London: Royal College of Nursing; 2002.

31. Vermandere M, De Lepeleire J, Smeet S, et al. Spirituality in general practice: a qualitative evidence synthesis. *British Journal of General Practice*. 2001; 749–760.

32. Stranahan S. Spiritual perception, attitudes about spiritual care, and spiritual care practices among nurse practitioners. *Western Journal of Nursing Research*. 2001; 23(1):90–104.

33. Ellis M, Campbell J. Patients' views about discussing spiritual issues with primary care physicians. *Southern Medical Journal*. 2004; 97(12):1158–1163.

34. Cummings J. *Compassion in Practice – Nursing Midwifery and Care Staff our Vision and Strategy*. London: NHS England; 2012.

35. Koenig H. Spirituality and mental health. *International Journal of Applied Psychoanalytical Studies*. 2010; 7:116–122.

36. Francis R. *Report of the Mid Staffordshire NHS Foundation Trust Public Inquiry*. Norwich: The Stationery Office; 2013.

37. Ballat J, Campling P. *Intelligent Kindness: Reforming the Culture of Healthcare*. London: Royal College of Psychiatrists; 2013.

38. Campling P. Reforming the culture of healthcare: the case for intelligent kindness, *British Journal of Psychiatry Bulletin*. 2015; 39:1–5.

39. Maltby J, Day L, Macaskill A. *Personality, Individual Difference and Intelligence* (2nd edition). Harlow: Pearson Education; 2010.

40. Hogg M, Vaughan G. *Social Psychology* (3rd edition). Harlow: Pearson Education; 2002.

41. Wright S. *Reflections on Spirituality and Health*. London: Whurr; 2005.

42. Wynne L. Spiritual care at the end of life. *Nursing Standard*. 2013; 28(2):41–45.

43. Tanyi R, McKenzie M, Chapek C. How family practice physicians, nurse practitioners and physician assistants incorporate spiritual care in practice. *Journal of the American Academy of Nurse Practitioners*. 2009; 21:690–697.

44. Venning P, Durie A, Roland C, Leese B. Randomised control trial cost effectiveness of general practitioners and nurse practitioners in primary care. *British Medical Journal*. 2000; 320:1048–1053.

45. Nursing and Midwifery Council. *The Code – Professional Standards of Practice and Behaviour for Nurses and Midwives*. London: NMC; 2015.

46. General Medical Council. *Personal Beliefs and Medical Practice*. London: General Medical Council; 2013.

47. Department of Health. *Liberating the NHS: No Decision about Me without Me*. London: Department of Health; 2012.

48. Royal College of Psychiatrists. Spirituality and mental health. Available at: http://www.rcpsych.ac.uk/mentalhealthinfo/treatments/spiritualityandmentalhealth.aspx (accessed 23/6/16).

49. Walters C, Edwards N. *Moving healthcare closer to home*. London: Monitor. 2013. Available at: https://www.gov.uk/government/uploads/system/uploads/attachment_data/file/459400/moving_healthcare_closer_to_home_summary.pdf (accessed 16/4/16).

Spiritual Teamwork within End of Life Care

10

Jonathan Sharp and Seamus Nash

Introduction

Spiritual awareness and praxis are, based on our professional and personal experiences, central aspects of current hospice care (1). This chapter explores the phenomenon of 'spiritual teamwork' within end of life care with reference to multi-disciplinary team (MDT) working within our place of employment – a 16-bed hospice located in West Yorkshire.

We hope to show what spiritual teamwork looks like in practice, with vignettes from our practice within the hospice and aided by illustrations from colleagues. Our premise is that spiritual teamwork is a holistic practice which is patient-centred. This means the patient is the *first* in the relationship and involves the worker being a responsive and available agent within the caring relationship. Central to the practice of spiritual teamwork is that the patient is perceived and engaged with *as a person,* who has worth, who is self-determining and who can take a key role in their own care. In essence, spiritual teamwork is based upon a spirituality of non-interference where the team members discern with the patient, with mindful compassion, the best course of action. Skills and attitudes essential to spiritual teamwork are empathy, active listening and attending skills, presence, genuineness and unconditional positive regard (see discussion in Chapter 1).

Although not academic in orientation and focus, we draw on instances from current literature to inform our discussion. Our aim is to offer a view of spiritual working and teamwork that is current and relevant to professionals in practice or to interested others.

Seamus Writes

I have been working in end of life care since 2005 and in social care since 1990. I originally was a scholastic in a Roman Catholic religious community and undertook formation training in London. I trained as a social worker then as a psychotherapist, finding that I had a natural ability to listen to people – which has usually been a source of joy and at times difficulty. In training as a client-centred psychotherapist, in the model advocated by Carl Rogers and his colleagues, I found a very real degree of freedom as the central tenet of client-, or as it is usually now called, 'person-centred' therapy is that 'the client knows best'. Although I personally believe in a 'God', I also acknowledge and value many cultural, spiritual and philosophical traditions. My psychotherapeutic practice is influenced also by encounter and dialogic forms of person-centred therapy; particularly the work of Schmid whom we cite here. In my practice, I attempt to offer an *anam cara* relationship – from the Celtic Christian construct meaning 'soul friend'. O'Donohue (2) wrote that the *anam cara* was the one to whom you sought to confess, to reveal the hidden intimacies of your life. The soul friend understands without judgement, allowing mask and pretensions to fall away and the person to experience that they are loved unconditionally. This is my 'calling' or vocation – it is a spiritually informed decision to *be* and *act* in this manner.

Jonathan Writes

As an ordained minister in the Methodist Church, I have a quarter of a century's experience of dealing with the rites of passage that mark, for the human person, entry into the world (Baptism), entry into an intimate and covenantal partnership with another person (Marriage), and departure from life on earth (Funeral). These are significant moments in the life not only of an individual but of a community; they are part of the discourse of that story which forms, encultures and is in turn shaped by each individual. It would be quite possible for me to deal with these rather as workers on the Ford Motor production line deal with bolting wheels onto Fiestas and Mondeos, to treat people as items to be processed along the conveyor belt of life, and thereby reduce, devalue and dehumanise … It *would* be quite possible, but would be at ethical odds to what I understand human beings to be. Human beings are not biomechanical machines to be processed dispassionately!

That, however, is just part of what informs my work as a practitioner of holistic and spiritual health care. I began working life at age 17 in Clinical Chemistry (Pathology) at a major Merseyside hospital. I pursued a career and studies as a biomedical scientist for a decade including several years in paediatrics where, besides collecting and analysing blood samples, I was involved in postgraduate research into the treatment of childhood leukaemias. From my late teens I have been immersed as a member of different teams in questions of what it is to be human, of meaning and purpose, of spiritual need and spiritual care …

After a decade in the NHS I was accepted for ordination training and for 17 years served churches in Cheshire and Yorkshire. My personal spirituality is eclectic – I share with Seamus in many aspects of this, especially the Celtic. My approach with interventions is largely Rogerian and thus person-centred. For the past decade I have been a whole-time health care chaplain firstly in acute medicine, now in palliative care.

My practice is to be led by the Other, to serve in a spiritually-informed way, because a chaplain is a minister and as Morris puts it, 'unless words have lost their meaning, a minister is simply one who is humanely useful' (3, p.14).

Defining Spirituality

Throughout the literature, there are numerous definitions of spirituality. In discussing these definitions, we feel that *spirituality* is that which gives a person worth, purpose and hope.

We recognise that 'Religion' is often conflated with spirituality but whilst religious belief may be a part of spirituality in its wider sense, we feel these are distinct if overlapping categories (4,5). Elkins (6) is clear, 'the spiritual is that which gives a person's life purpose, meaning and value. It *may* include a religious dimension but does not have to' (our emphasis).

Spiritual Teamwork

We propose the following definition of *spiritual teamwork* as working and being part of a team which works in a holistic and spiritually informed manner, putting the patient and their experiences at the centre of our work, respecting and upholding their dignity and right to self-determination, offering them unconditional positive regard, warmth, care and compassion.

Central to the practice of spiritual teamwork within our hospice, is the concept of *vocation*, 'A strong feeling of suitability for a particular career or occupation … a person's employment or main occupation, especially regarded as worthy and requiring dedication' (7).

'Vocation' comes from the Latin *vocare*, 'to call' (7). When talking with colleagues about spiritual teamwork, and hospice working in general, they describe feeling 'called' to the work they do, they 'believe' in the work; colleagues wish to be 'human' with patients, to treat patients and their families with 'love', 'care' and respect'. Working in this manner, therefore, is a *spiritually informed decision*.

For us, the ideas of Levinas (8) form the bedrock of our concept of spiritual teamwork. Levinas writes that the 'Other' (the patient, client: Person) calls or 'signals' us as professional workers to respond to their call. In a real sense the 'Other' (the patient, client) *calls* us into relationship with them. Spiritual teamwork is thus conceived and perceived as a 'Thou–I' relationship. The patient calls and the worker responds. It is the *worker's response-ability* to the 'call' of the Other which begins spiritual teamwork.

Spiritual teamwork has its philosophical roots in a *phenomenological approach*. The word 'phenomenon' comes from the Greek. In its active form its means 'show, bring to light, make appear, *announce*'; in passive voice it means 'be shown, come to light, appear, *come into being*'. According to Schmid (9), an approach is phenomenological if the direction, the *movement*, goes *from the patient to the worker*: the client 'shows and announces'. This is exactly the Thou–I relationship of Levinas (8).

Schmid (9), citing Rogers, feels that the worker thus encounters the patient 'person to person'. *Presence* is the fundamental way of 'being together', the existential foundation of the person-centred therapy's core conditions (9,10). For Schmid this relating is possible only from a 'We-perspective', hence he feels Presence is:

- Co-operation arising out of co-existence
- Co-responding (to given experiencings) out of co-experiencing
- Co-creating out of (in its best moments mutual) encounter (11)

Colleagues feel that being present, available and focused affords and affirms the patient's *dignity* and self of worth. Chochinov's (12, p.1) research supports the view that 'the basic tenets of palliative care may be summarized as the goal of helping patients to die with dignity'.

Finally, spiritual teamwork also elicits the abilities of members of the MDT to be with and to *journey with* the patient/client for however brief a period; offering care, compassion, and being hopeful with and for them. As mentioned, 'spiritual non-interference' and support of the patient are paramount. The MDT then do not *set up* the discourse within their work; rather they take their cues from the patient who allows the MDT to enter into their world. Intervention is an *invitation* and *working with* not an *imposition*. Therefore, spiritual teamwork is not necessarily focused primarily on goals, skills or interventionist approaches firstly, but on building a *relationship* with a real human person.

Exploring the Concept of the 'Image' of the Human Being

In our experience, social and health care practice does give weight to the concept of treating patient/clients/service users as *persons*. The terms 'person-centred care' and 'patient-centred care' are so rooted in the discourse of the helping professions that they are readily accepted without much reflection of what is actually being implied. Services are proud to announce themselves as 'person/patient-centred'.

Whilst this is indeed laudable, upon closer examination, the terms, and to a certain extent the discourse, around patient/person-centred care hold a profound challenge to those of us engaged in professional care across disciplines. The term 'person-centred' originates from the work of Carl Rogers (13–16) and his associates from the psychotherapy and counselling world. Rogers (17) first used the term 'client' in response to the expert-led practices of his time and emphasising that it is the client's experiencing – not the therapist's expertise, nor diagnosis, which is central.

Building on client-centred psychotherapy and humanistic philosophy and practice we perceive the core of spiritual teamwork is centred on the *image of the human being* which the hospice movement and our own MDT seeks to support. The 'patient' or 'client' is first and foremost related to as a whole *person* who we relate to and treat in a *person-to-person* manner. We concur with Schmid (18) that this ethical and anthropological stance means we are bound to then only act in ways that always uphold this basic relationship, and to promote independence and dignity.

'What is a human being?' Your answer to this question gives a clue to how you view and construct what it is to be a 'human being'. All theories of helping hold a view of what it is to be human including assumptions concerning how human beings are (what their nature is, their essence, their peculiarity, their meaning of life, etc.), how they develop, how they get into trouble and how they can be helped. Schmid asserts 'related questions are, for example, whether humans are free or not (and thus responsible or not), whether they are good or evil.

Images of the human being have the following characteristics:

- They are models (representations of ideas of a typological nature).
- They represent, select and construct 'reality' (i.e. they are not reality itself).
- They have a heuristic function (they help to find new perspectives).

- They serve as guidelines for practice.
- Most important, they are trans-empirical (they are basic *beliefs* – they cannot be proved)' (9).

Informed by our beliefs and training, any approach to helping is person-centred if it regards the human being as a person and acts accordingly on a person-to-person basis (9). These are central tenets of spiritually informed teamwork that we now advocate and act upon. This now informs the question of what person/patient-centred helping is. It is built on certain epistemological, anthropological, ethical and ontological assumptions of what it is to be human. These assumptions that inform spiritual teamwork *necessarily preclude* working in a way that labels and objectifies the patient/person. They motivate the worker to act in certain ways – to be non-controlling, upholding dignity and self-determination, to be non-judgmental and to be loving and compassionate.

What Is a *Person-Centred* Image of the Human Being?

Schmid (11) writes that human beings are characterized as persons if they are denoted in their unique individuality, worth and dignity (the substantial notion of being a person), as well as their other interconnectedness, being-from and being-towards others (relational conception of becoming a person). Being a person requires both autonomy and solidarity, both sovereignty and commitment. According to Schmid, the founder of client-centred psychotherapy Carl Rogers, combined both views in a unique way for psychotherapy.

Schmid writes that person-centred personality and relationship theory understands 'personalization' as a process of becoming independent *and* of developing relationships.

Thus from Schmid we can understand 'helping' as *both* enabling personality development *and* encounter person to person, 'the practice is characterized by *presence* – which means a principled non-directivity and empathic positive regard as a way of being 'with' the client, *together with* a position 'counter' the client, i.e. a committed 'en-counter' as a person meeting the Other face to face' (18, pp. 74–90).

Schmid sums up thus:

> If this is the underlying image of the human being, then the distinguishing characteristics of a *person*-centred approach can be stated in the following three short sentences.
>
> 1. Client and therapist spring from a fundamental 'We'.
> 2. The client comes first.
> 3. The therapist is present.
>
> Yet these seemingly simple statements imply a revolutionary change of paradigms (20, p.2).

We begin work together in a *We*. Schmid writes beautifully as he says 'None of us came to us from the outside; everyone was born within and into this We. If we ignore this, we ignore that we are unavoidably a part of the world; we ignore our roots, our past, present and future; there is no 'en-counter'' (19). Consequently, then, the entire spiritual teamwork approach would become unrealistic and thus naïve: we are all some else's Other.

Being on 'the Receiving End'

For some people receiving institutionalised health-care their experience is very much like being a commodity processed in a factory. Winbolt-Lewis (20) quotes one 80-year-old person: 'I felt like a packet of biscuits being hurled from one place to another ... I never thought that I would one day be known simply as a patient number...'.

Caring and Concern = Compassion = Spiritual Care

Caring for others consists in expressing love in 'practical action'. This means ensuring that staff acknowledge the patient or client's situation, ensuring necessary nutrition and hydration, welcoming and befriending, providing appropriate clothing and shelter, tending to the sick and so forth. These actions show that a person is accorded worth, dignity and respect; these actions demonstrate that the recipient has value simply for who they are; and they make manifest the givers' values and intentions as regards their belief in what it is to be human and how other humans ought to be treated. Colleagues often report that if they are allowed the necessary time and space to care for the patient, *according to their perceived vocation*, they then really feel they are 'doing their job'. Handzo and Koenig (21) state: 'In relating ... as a caring human being to another human being who needs help, we are giving spiritual care.'

Speck (22) offers a corrective to the perceived 'medical model' of health care with its emphasis on a technological approach designed to eradicate disease rather than treat the whole person. He notes a new 'emphasis on holistic medicine with its focus on the person who has the sickness rather than the sickness itself'. In other words, this is spiritual care at work in 'giving the person back to the patient' (20); namely treating the patient as a *human being.*

As Cassidy declares, compassion is 'to enter into the suffering of another' (23, p.5). Thus, Compassionate Care is to walk with people in the midst of their pain, to go with them along their lonely and frightening road, sharing their darkness. Such activity puts the accompanier in a place of vulnerability.

A hospital chaplain reflects on a particularly difficult pastoral encounter – an 8-month-old child had died, and describes his feelings: 'I did not come bringing any sort of expertise. The only thing I had to offer was me. One person coming alongside some others' (24). This chaplain clearly felt exceedingly vulnerable.

And yet, 'Vulnerability is the birthplace of connection and the path to the feeling of worthiness. If it doesn't feel vulnerable, the sharing is probably not constructive' (25). Green writes creatively about the coming alongside another, about the mutual vulnerability being the birthplace of connection, and about the entering of a shared liminal space pregnant with the possibility of becoming. He references Jung: 'The meeting of two personalities is like the contact of two chemical substances: if there is any reaction, both are transformed' (26, p.18).

Whorton's research confirms that this is borne out by the experience of those accompanied, 'Those who encourage us most are those who can look us in the eye and see through to our soul, and seeing what is there still reach out their hand to us. They stay with us, and their staying with us means we can stay with the journey too' (27, p.123).

The chaplain may be vulnerable or feel vulnerable, but she is still the health care professional who will leave the hospice and travel home for tea. So what kind of vulnerability is it? We offer two responses. Firstly, Kelly (28):

> ... in supporting others at times of loss and transition, can I wait with, own and allow to be, my helplessness as well as other peoples? Undoubtedly, the ability to provide others with a 'non-anxious presence' in their time of uncertainty or transition is central to the provision of sensitive pastoral and spiritual care.

This is not just the work of the spiritual care team, and indeed the provision of a 'non-anxious presence' by other staff and volunteers of the MDT working in a spiritually informed way is *precisely* the comforting key that opens the way to more profound spiritual encounter and soul-work.

Secondly, Perryman's response (29) to the hospital chaplain's account (24) of his difficult pastoral encounter criticises it as disingenuous on the grounds that, 'He did at least eight things which were possible only because he had sophisticated training and considerable experience in theology, pastoral care, priesthood and chaplaincy.'

As previously, our experience convinces us that such spiritual care intervention, the chaplain's presencing and acting, are made possible by the whole MDT (staff and volunteers) working in a spiritually informed way.

Spiritual Care

Spiritual Care is defined variously within the literature. For example, Cressy and Winbolt-Lewis (30) argue that 'Spiritual care conveys to the patients that they have value and are loved simply for who they are, regardless of their illness, colour or creed and it can be given by any carer whatever their rank or profession. All good caring is spiritual.'

Julia Neuberger (31, p.7), affirming the valuable contribution towards spiritual care made by each member of the MDT, states:

> But in fact spiritual care goes much wider than chaplaincy. It is not only chaplains who provide it. It is not even primarily chaplains who provide it. It can, and often is, provided by every member of the health care team, if they have the sensitivity and skills, as well as other staff members, particularly the cleaning (and domestic or housekeeping) and portering staff, who often, by their very common sense and willingness to talk where health care staff fear to tread, provide some of the best spiritual care in our health care settings in this country.

Alternatively, Walter (32), with a specific view towards end of life care, questions the 'assumption in palliative care literature ... that all patients have a spiritual dimension and that all staff can offer spiritual care.' Walter is critical of the discourses that abound within the broader health care system around 'spiritual care' and raises valid points: spiritually informed practice may indeed come more easily to some colleagues than to others.

Whilst we share his concerns, we also write from our experience within a strong MDT who have all contributed to the growth in 'spiritual care' and to related policies within the hospice-the team believes its work is spiritual as well as nursing, doctoring, social working and so on. Spiritual teamwork is a reality; it is fuelled by vocation and grounded in treating patients as human beings rather than sets of complex diagnoses. One of the bedrocks of our ethos is, in our Medical Director's words, that we strive for the hospice ethos and practice to be 'flexible around patient needs, not the patient to be flexible around our systems' (33).

We also are concerned by the view that spiritual care is hard to define, or is too cumbersome. In our work, it simply means demonstrating love, concern and compassion in a person-centred way. It is standing shoulder to shoulder with the patient and the family facing the impending event of dying and death.

We concur with Gordon et al (34, p.2) that for us, in a real sense 'all people, regardless of their life stance have an innate spirituality.' Spirituality may indeed be individual to each person, but every encounter therefore implies the confluence of two spiritualities.

Context and Delivery

At the hospice we are working within end of life care. The context is important as these are often patients' last days. With them the MDT carry hope for and often with them (35).

The delivery of spiritual care is an interpersonal activity; it requires relationship. It is not a discreet *I-Thou* transaction, but a *We* interaction (36). Schmid (19) describes how 'response-ability is the basic category of being a person: Out of encounter arises the obligation to respond.' That response 'means service to the person out of solidarity' (19, p.2).

Spiritual Teamwork is Spiritual Journeying and Accompaniment

Many religions have a tradition of pilgrimage or journeying with others. There is much to be learned by the health care team about cooperative journeying with patients and their families. As spiritual caregivers we often find ourselves 'playing in the margins of meaning' (37). Let us be clear here. The content of this 'playing' is exactly meaning-making, even the reconstructing of meaning in the face of the traumatic, dramatic instability caused by a terminal diagnosis. Here again, spiritually-informed presencing and work begins with drawing alongside a person and accompanying compassionately in solidarity. Spiritual teamwork is cooperative, giver and receiver both being vulnerable and open to the possibility of change and growth – 'we do, we struggle to make meaning and share' (38, p.3).

Secondly, and holding to the image of journeying through what may seem a dusty wilderness, once engagement is made and the beginnings of a therapeutic relationship established, the spiritual care-giver is entering upon what Jonathan describes as 'the adventure of the unrehearsed critical conversation'.

Again, spiritual care 'often is provided by every member of the health care team' (31) and Schmid (19) makes the point that in such institutions and therapeutic disciplines that focus on individualised care, 'we need distinction and we need cooperation.' There are many kinds of roles, but they are complementary. Gordon et al (34, p.3) express this well: 'a health care practitioner's humanity, the self, is the most effective therapeutic tool that they possess.'

Role of Chaplain/Spiritual Care Coordinator

Caring presence and presencing often appear in the nursing literature as special ways of 'being there' or 'being with' another (39). To 'presence oneself' with another person means making oneself available to understand and be with another. 'Presencing' may be understood as the situating of the spiritual care team (paid and volunteer) member's self sensitively and imaginatively in the world of those being cared for. 'Presencing' is the gift of oneself in human interaction and requires receiving another's presence as well as giving one's presence. By caring for and valuing the other, the spiritual care team member's own being is enhanced.

We note again the comment from Haig (24) that in the exercise of spiritual care 'the only thing I had to offer was myself' (*cf* 27, p.5).

Cressy and Winbolt-Lewis (30) aver that

> … spiritual care conveys to people that they have value and are loved simply for who they are regardless of their colour or creed, health, wealth, education or sexuality, and it can be given by any carer whatever their rank or profession. All good caring is spiritual.
>
> The spiritual dimension refers to 'a quality that goes beyond religious affiliation, that strives for inspirations, reverence, awe, meaning and purpose' … .
>
> Spiritual care, offered by anyone in the health care team is a gesture of love, and we agree with Morris, that 'love requires no medium, no wire or gadgets, nor paper or print. Only one thing is necessary: bare presence, touchability' (40, p.28).

So,

> Quality care has to do with the direct interaction of care between receiver and care-giver. A caring act becomes spiritual when it comes from the heart and addresses the total needs of the patient and not just the 'part'. This quality of empathic engagement is a prime feature of spiritual care, providing aliveness and health (30, p.3).

Vignettes

MDT Staff members spoke to us regarding this chapter and some offered the following vignettes as examples of spiritual teamwork.

Thank You Cards

A young middle-aged man on the in patient unit (IPU) knew that his time was short, and although he wanted to compose and self-pen some cards for relatives and special friends to say 'thank you' for their touch on his life, he knew that his energy levels were waning and he had insufficient resources for the combination of mental focus and fine motor control required. Bernadette, the hospice therapy assistant who supports occupational and physiotherapists, patiently and sensitively over a period of days helped the gentleman find the words and then wrote the cards for him, the gentleman himself signing them. In conversation with me, he expressed his gratitude for Bernadette's time and helpfulness.

Very soon after completing the cards, the gentleman died. Whilst speaking with the funeral director I was told that she'd heard from the family about how they were 'blown away' by what the man had written, and how moved and grateful they were.

Bernadette played a major role in helping this person explore and express his deepest feelings. Her work with him positively facilitated his negotiating of his last days of life and will also aid the grief journeys of those bereaved.

This is a wonderful example of spiritual and emotional support.

Wi-Fi

'Terry? I've just come to thank you for the wonderful spiritual care you've exercised in room 3', I said to the hospice information technology (IT) Manager.

'Pardon?!' came the puzzled reply, accompanied by raised eyebrows.

'Room 3. You sorted the wi-fi connection out'.

'Ye-e-e-es …' still puzzled.

'That's spiritual care. Good job! Well done!'

Shake of bemused head.

'You set up the wi-fi signal so that patient's son, who lives in Dorset, and whose work requires daily global communication, could bring his laptop into the hospice room and work from there. He can carry on working – thus reducing his anxieties and making him feel he's still making a positive contribution; he can also be present with his father, fostering their intimate emotional/spiritual bond. His father has the close company of his son. That's incredibly special, life-affirming and life-enhancing. And made possible by the wi-fi signal *you* organised'.

Leaning Over the Edge

I walked into the four-bed bay that this week was populated by men. I greeted Colin and asked how he was this day. 'Do you want to step outside?' he asked, gesturing with his head to the exterior door in the corner. 'Sure.'

We walked slowly out onto the decking that surrounds the hospice and affords wonderful views of the landscaped grounds, and we leant against the safety rail to peer over.

I knew from the morning multidisciplinary team handover meetings that one of the medics had had to be upfront about Colin's prognosis. It was this that was on his mind. The words came out slowly:

'I had a bit of a hard word the other day. I knew I didn't have a very long time, but I was hoping for maybe another year …

'That young doctor, she told me that it's more like 3 months …

And I want to stay here … but she says I can't because the care I need can be provided elsewhere now … nursing home …

Thing is … I've got to tell my children and my mum … and I shan't be able to until Saturday, and that's 4 days, and mum doesn't know but her brother's got cancer, too, and he's told me but asked me not tell her …

She was so patient and gentle with me – that young doctor.

She almost knelt by my bed … made sure I could see her face … and really took her time to make sure I understood … and that I could see … '

And it went momentarily quiet except for the quiet hum of traffic and the chirps and twitters of birds in the gardens

'I could see that it was costing her to tell me …

I really felt for her. She had to be so brave …

Where do people like that get that from?'

It took me about three days to catch that doctor in a quiet moment, by which time Colin's mum had visited and he'd been able to say to me with a smile that 'It turns out mum knew more than I thought … '.

But find her I did. And fed back to her what Colin had said. And reminded her that it was clear that how she had spoken had come from her heart. She'd done a very, very difficult thing with incredible sensitivity, compassion and respect, and at no little cost to herself.

Memories in Future Tense

Jane had been attending Support & Therapy at hospice for about 10 months. She tended to sit quietly in the main lounge area. Gradually, through her gentle presence, Rachel, the activities support worker, began to get Jane to engage. Jane's main anxiety was for her 14-year-old daughter and how she would feel growing up without her mum.

Rachel disclosed something of her own life journey, sharing soul-learning from her own experience – her own mum had died when Rachel was 34, and her mum's mum died when her mum was 64. Rachel gently told Jane, 'It doesn't matter whether your daughter is 14, 24, 34 or 64, the impact will still be the same … the questions you've not asked, the simple things, like what time I was born, how much I weighed when I was born … It doesn't matter what age you are, there's always a question'.

Rachel persuaded Jane into the Art Room and encouraged her to bring in something of significance. Jane brought a shell that her daughter had found. It was a kind of clam that when opened looked like wings. Jane chose a gem from the items Rachel brought out, and glued it between the hinges of the shell – and it became an angel with wings.

During this time in the art room, Rachel disclosed more of her own experience – she has all the cards her mum ever sent her, including for her own first pregnancy, and a card her mum wrote for Rachel's daughter's birthday even though she didn't live to see it. Rachel's mum had also written her a letter before she died (in the very hospice this encounter is taking place) and Rachel treasures this and reads it again and again and 'every time I read it, I can hear her saying it. It's my most cherished thing in the world'.

'So, Jane, let's not dwell on the past, let's make a future … '

Over the weeks, Jane has been preparing everything she wants to do for her daughter – cards for exams, driving lessons, engagement, wedding, and for boy and girl babies …

Rachel is self-deprecating; she describes this as simply 'doing what I'm meant to do' … This is beautifully spiritually-informed vocational work.

… One More Lovely Thing*

An auxiliary nurse reflects – A patient who was on her second admission to hospice came up to the nurses' station after saying goodnight to her husband and said, 'I hope you will not mind what I have to say and you will take it as the compliment it is meant to be. I have noticed you have what can only be described as an air of serenity about you. Whenever you enter a room or speak to a patient, the atmosphere immediately becomes more calm and relaxed. I have racked my brain to find who it is that you remind me of, both in looks and serenity, and it is the Mother Superior from *The Sound of Music*. The way she deals with all Maria's problems in a calm, gentle and reassuring way and leaves a sense of peace wherever she goes.'

The auxiliary was greatly encouraged by this, recognising that, in her own words, 'no matter how small a part we play we can make a difference to someone's quality of life and their journey to the end'.

The spiritual care coordinator observes that in this instance, as in many, the patients themselves (as well as their relatives and carers) are actively engaged in the spiritually informed work that makes the hospice a nursery of nurture for vulnerable lives (the staff included).

Supporting staff in their own development and skills is essential to considering and providing excellent spiritual teamwork. At hospice we provide the following, which is not exhaustive:

- Clinical and non-clinical supervision groups
- Management support
- Staff well-being policy
- Informal staff support
- Extensive training and personal development opportunities
- Critical incident de-briefs when necessary
- Skills training in advanced listening skills and communication
- Spiritual care training
- Appraisals

Summary of Spiritual Teamworking

Neuberger's assertion that *all* members of the health care team, whether staff or volunteers, 'if they have the sensitivity and skills … provide some of the best spiritual care' (30), is extremely valid. To the spiritual care team they afford immeasurable assistance in creating the supportive atmosphere and safe environment in which soul-work may take place (*cf* 26, p.xiii). And, as Vanstone asserts

---

* *The Sound of Music*, lyric: Oscar Hammerstein II.

… assistance is a very physical word: it denotes putting one's body somewhere, giving one's physical presence to someone and the gift of one's physical presence is, in a sense, unique: it cannot be wholly or adequately replaced by any other gift or any other means of communication (41, p.118).

Relationship-building – that is, getting to know the person – is essential to achieving the best outcome for the patient. Therefore, as Luker et al (42) assert, establishing early contact and 'knowing the patient' become linked with high-quality palliative care.

Cooper (35) suggests that … a 'sense of connectedness is fostered by the use of presence, active listening and demonstration of compassion.'

What is true for relationships and interactions with patients and relatives is equally true for relationships within the health care team. A Christian chaplain may see this in terms of *Ephesians 4*, in which the gifts given to the people (*aka* the skill sets, competencies and expertise of the MDT) are for the building up of the body of people, said body being called to live and be so that all others may have life in all its fullness.

To this end (i.e. the building up of the body of the MDT and equipping each member for the work in hand), a significant element of spiritual care is staff support, both formally and informally. The family care team and spiritual care team are involved in facilitating clinical supervision for groups and individuals and providing learning opportunities at induction for new members of staff (paid and volunteer), and for continuing staff and volunteers in such areas as spirituality, grief and loss, ageing and spirituality, and the spiritual cost of bereavement.

Supporting staff in their own development and skills is essential to providing excellent spiritual teamwork.

There is a comprehensive module of training for new volunteers on the spiritual care team, and there is collaborative work with other members of the MDT in facilitating placement opportunities for clergy-in-training from the local theological college. There is also regular interaction with and input to the town interfaith forum. Much informal work, through presencing and the practical truth that the 'corridors are our cloisters', gently nurtures the life of the body and its individual members.

In the words of the hymn *The Servant Song*:

> We are pilgrims on a journey,
> and companions on the road;
> we are here to help each other
> walk the mile and bear the load (43).

Commenting on those very words, from the hymn above, and out of his own experience as hospice chaplain, Whorton (44, p.123) writes, 'those who encourage us most are those who can look us in the eye and see through to our soul, and seeing what is there still reach out their hand to us. They stay with us, and their staying with us means we can stay with the journey too.'

In end of life care there are some things we can help with and some we cannot, things we can fix and many we cannot, and plenty of ways in which we can serve the needs of individuals and the institution. Overall, the ethos and practice of the whole MDT is to serve, for as Remen (45) notes, 'Helping, fixing, and serving represent three different ways of seeing life. When you help, you see life as weak. When you fix, you see life as broken. When you serve, you see life as whole. Fixing and helping may be the work of the ego, and service the work of the soul'.

Conclusion: Characterising Spiritual Teamwork as a Spiritual, Ethical and Political Stance

The characterizing fundamental statements explaining a genuinely spiritual teamwork and indeed a *person*-centred approach can now be formulated:

1. Patient and MDT co-operate on the basis of a fundamental 'We', which constitutes their person to person relationships.
2. The patient comes first, because he or she is the expert.
3. The MDT responds to the client's call by being Present (9).

References

1. Holloway M, Adamson S, McSherry W, Swinton J. Spiritual care at the end of life: a systematic review of the literature. 2011. London: Department of Health. Available at: gov.uk/government/uploads/system/uploads/attachment_data/file/215798/dh_123804.pdf (accessed 7/6/16).
2. O'Donohue J. *Anam Cara: Wisdom from the Celtic World*. London: Bantam Press; 1997.
3. Morris C. *Include Me Out*. London: Epworth; 1968.
4. Kelly E. Preparation for providing spiritual care. *Scottish Journal of Healthcare Chaplaincy*. 2002; 5(2): 11.
5. Robinson S, Kendrick K, Brown A. *Spirituality and the Practice of Healthcare*. London: Palgrave MacMillan; 2003.
6. Elkins DN, Hedstrom LJ, Hughes LL, Leaf JA, Saunders C. Toward a humanistic-phenomenological spirituality: definition, description, and measurement. *Journal of Humanistic Psychology*. 1988; 28(4): 5–18.
7. Oxford University Press. Oxford English Dictionary. Available at: oed.com/view/Entry/224289?redirected From=vocation#eid (accessed 27/6/16).
8. Levinas E. *Totality and Infinity: An Essay on Exteriority*. Pittsburgh PA: Duquesne University Press; 1969.
9. Schmid PF. The characteristics of a person-centred approach to therapy and counselling: criteria for identity and coherence. Carl Rogers Symposium; 2002; July 27.
10. Schmid PF. Acknowledgement: the art of responding. Dialogical and ethical perspectives on the challenge of unconditional personal relationships in therapy and beyond. In Bozarth J, Wilkins P (eds). *Unconditional Positive Regard*. Ross-on-Wye: PCCS Books; 2001, pp 49–64.
11. Schmid PF. The necessary and sufficient conditions of being person-centred: on identity, integrity, integration and differentiation of the paradigm. In Watson JC, Goldman R, Warner MS (eds). *Client-Centred and Experiential Psychotherapy in the 21st Century*. Ross-on-Wye: PCCS Books; 2002, pp 36–51.
12. Chochinov, HM. Dignity conserving care - a new model for palliative care. *Journal of the American Medical Association*. 2010; 287(17). Available at: http://jama.jamanetwork.com/article.aspx?articleid=194871 (accessed 7/6/16).
13. Rogers C. *Client Centred Therapy*. London: Constable; 1951.
14. Rogers C. The necessary and sufficient conditions of therapeutic personality change. *Journal of Consulting Psychotherapy*. 1957; 21(95): 103.
15. Rogers C. A theory of therapy, personality and interpersonal relationships, as developed in the client-centred framework. In Koch S (ed). *A Study of Science 3. Formulations of the Person and the Social Context*. New York: McGraw Hill; 1959; pp 184–246.
16. Rogers C. *On Becoming a Person: A Therapist's View of Therapy*. London: Constable; 1961.

17. Rogers C. *Counselling and Psychotherapy*. Boston: Houghton Mifflin; 1942.

18. Schmid PF. On becoming a person-centred approach: a person-centred understanding of the person. In Thorne B, Lambers E (eds). *Person-Centred Therapy: A European Perspective*. London: Sage; 1998, pp 38–90.

19. Schmid PF. The unavoidable We in therapy. Carl Rogers Symposium; 2002; July 25.

20. Winbolt-Lewis M. The Mid-Yorkshire Hospitals NHS Trust chaplaincy holistic and spiritual healthcare policy. Wakefield: Mid-Yorkshire Hospitals NHS Trust; 2011.

21. Handzo G, Koenig HG. Spiritual care: whose job is it anyway? *Southern Medical Journal*. 2004; 97(12): 1242–1244.

22. Speck P. *Being There: Pastoral Care in Time of Illness*. London: SPCK; 1988.

23. Cassidy, S. *Sharing The Darkness*. London: Darton, Longman and Todd; 1988.

24. Haig A. Sermon. *Journal of Healthcare Chaplaincy*. 2010; 10(1): 3–8

25. Brene, B. Vulnerability. Available at: brainyquote.com/quotes/authors/b/brene_brown.html (accessed 14/5/2016).

26. Green R. *Only Connect: Worship and Liturgy from the Perspective of Pastoral Care*. London: Darton, Longman and Todd; 1987.

27. Whorton B. *Reflective Caring: Imaginative Listening to Pastoral Experience*. London: SPCK; 2011.

28. Kelly E. *Personhood and Presence: Self as a Resource for Spiritual Care*. London: Bloomsbury; 2014.

29. Perryman J. Letter. *Journal of Healthcare Chaplaincy*. 2011; 11(1): 85–87.

30. Cressy R, Winbolt-Lewis M. *The Forgotten Heart of Care: A Model of Spiritual Care for the NHS*. Wakefield: Pinderfields and Pontefract Hospitals NHS Trust; 1999.

31. Neuberger J. Foreword. In Cobb M, Robshaw M (eds). *The Spiritual Challenge of Healthcare*. London: Churchill Livingstone; 1988.

32. Walter T. Spirituality in palliative care: opportunity or burden? *Palliative Medicine*. 2002; 16(2): 133–140.

33. Oxberry SG. What Does Kirkwood Do? Huddersfield: Kirkwood Hospice; 2015 (unpublished power point presentation, December, 2015).

34. Gordon T, Kelly E, Mitchell D. *Spiritual Care for Healthcare Professionals: Reflecting on Clinical Practice*. London: Radcliffe; 2011.

35. Cooper PG. The influence of hope on the psychosocial experience. In Carroll-Johnson RM, Gorman L, Bush NJ (eds). *Psychosocial Nursing Care Along the Cancer Continuum*. Pittsburgh PA: Oncology Nursing Society; 2000, pp 53–202.

36. Nolan S. *Spiritual Care at the End of Life: The Chaplain as 'Hopeful Presence'*. London: Jessica Kingsley; 2012.

37. Neelands J, Goode T. Playing in the margins of meaning: the ritual aesthetic in community performance. *Drama Australia Journal* 2008; 32(1): 82.

38. Owens A, Barber K. *Dramaworks: Successful Drama Pretexts Across the Age Range*. Carlisle: Carel; 1996.

39. Nelms TP. Living a caring presence in nursing: a Heideggerian hermeneutical anlysis. *Journal of Advanced Nursing*. 1996; 24(2): 368–374.

40. Morris C. *Wrestling with an Angel*. London: Fount; 1990.

41. Vanstone. *Fare Well in Christ*. London: Darton Longman and Todd; 1997.

42. Luker KA, Austin L, Caress A, Hallett CE. The importance of 'knowing the patient': community nurses' constructions of quality in providing palliative care. *Journal of Advanced Nursing*. 2000; 31(4): 775–782

43. Gillard R (ed). *The Servant Song. Singing the Faith*. London: Methodist Publishing; 2011, p. 611.

44. Whorton B. *Voices from the Hospice: Staying with Life Through Suffering and Waiting*. London: SCM; 2015.

45. Remen RM. HelpingFixingServing. 2016. Available at: uc.edu/content/dam/uc/honors/docs/communityengagement/HelpingFixingServing.pdf (accessed 14/5/2016).

Creative Organisations: Spirituality and Creativity in a Health Setting

11

Phil Walters, Steven Michael and Mike Gartland

Context

South West Yorkshire Partnership NHS Foundation Trust (SWYFT) provides general inpatient and community mental health and learning disability services as well as substance misuse services to over one million people across Barnsley, Calderdale, Kirklees and Wakefield. It provides forensic mental health services to the wider area of Yorkshire and Humber in the North of England.

In early 2001 a major review concerning mental health service configuration was undertaken in the Yorkshire region. The review team recommended the creation of a specialist mental health organisation to provide services to the localities of Calderdale, Kirklees and Wakefield, as well as act as a host for regional medium secure services. In 2002 South West Yorkshire Mental Health NHS Trust (SWYMHT), the predecessor organisation to SWYFT, came into being.

Despite facing significant financial challenges, from the outset SWYMHT sought to make the partnership with service users and carers central to all organisational development. Accordingly, significant engagement work was undertaken to ensure the organisation could build a strong shared value base upon which a clear service offer could be developed.

This sense of shared values became a touchstone for all future planning work. Also, at this time the Trust benefitted from having a clear steer in terms of national policy and associated implementation guidance. Although somewhat variable from locality to locality, there was further investment in mental health and learning disability services to support developments. However, policy directives alone cannot lead to a fully holistic service being offered to service users and carers; they need to be implemented by people. The sense of continued emphasis on every dimension of a person's life began to open up thinking as to how elements of spirituality and creativity could enhance the experience of people using the Trust's services. Despite the need to deliver on key policy requirements and achieve a stronger financial footing, the organisation made a deliberate choice to invest in areas such as pastoral and spiritual care and creative partnerships. This began on a small scale but has grown substantially over the years.

In 2006 a decision was taken by the Trust Board to make a formal application to become a Foundation Trust (1). The reasons for this were complex and multi-faceted. However, at the heart of the application lay a belief in the power of investing ownership and associated governance in the public and partner membership. Coupled with this was the opportunity to secure financial freedom to invest potential surplus generated into areas where real value could be added to the service offer, including innovative approaches to spirituality and creativity in health care.

Foundation Trust status was secured in 2009. Although a significant emphasis was placed on achieving a position of financial viability and sustainability, the commitment to developing a more holistic approach remained undiminished.

In the subsequent 2 years further engagement work was undertaken with service users, carers and staff to determine what should be the core purpose of the organisation over its next phase of development. Discussions took place with over 2500 people, and the feedback received was extremely consistent and led to the agreement of a core statement of purpose, often referred to as the Mission Statement: 'Enable people to reach their potential and to live well in their community'.

This renewed sense of purpose gave greater legitimacy to the developing approaches concerning both spirituality and creativity. Rather than being viewed purely as a provider of care and treatment, the Trust took a view that it should occupy a much stronger enabling function which was supportive of the agreed mission. Increasingly, service users, carers and staff reported favourably on their experiences in terms of finding a greater meaning for their life and work through initiatives driven by the spirituality and creativity agendas.

Spirit in Mind and Creative Minds, as they have become to be known, now occupy a strong and well-recognised place within the organisation's offer of services. A challenge still exists, however, in that it is difficult to provide comprehensive quantitative evidence to support their efficacy, particularly in a system where there is positivist orthodoxy in relation to what constitutes best evidence. Nonetheless, as the work has progressed there is a growing body of mainly qualitative evidence, based on the personal testimonies and narratives of service users and carers. There is great power in such narratives, some of which have been made into short films that can be found on the Creative Minds section of the SWYFT website (2). Both Spirit in Mind and Creative Minds have attracted significant national and international attention and recognition. This includes Creative Minds and Spirit in Mind presentations at the two Microsystems Festivals in Jonkoping, Sweden in February 2014 and 2015. Creative Minds also presented at the Co-producing and Co-delivering Recovery: Implementing Recovery through Organsational Change (ImROC) Conference in Yorkshire in March 2014 and has been recognised in the following national awards: *Health Service Journal*, Compassionate Patient Care Award, 2014; The Patient Experience Network, Strengthening the Foundation Award, 2014 and Building Better Healthcare Awards Best Collaborative Art Project, 2015.

Whether the organisational conditions which have supported such initiatives to date can be maintained remains to be seen, but the importance of telling the story to-date cannot be underestimated.

Case Study 1: Spirit in Mind

A health care project to develop partnerships between faith based organisations and the statutory sector was launched in West Yorkshire in 2015. Spirit in Mind brings together SWYFT and religious organisations such as churches and mosques in collaborative responses to areas of shared social concern. This may also include non-faith and humanist organisations. We also have a strong partnership with the University of Huddersfield, in particular their Spirituality Special Interest Group which has brought academic thinking to the approach. As such Spirit in Mind is part of a larger social movement reflected in recent government planning and legislation. Issues relating to religion and faith have received an increased level of attention from central government. Notable examples are the inclusion of Religion and Belief in the 2010 Equality Act (3) and initiatives on volunteering, prevention of violent extremism, community cohesion and empowerment (4). An ongoing climate of financial austerity has given additional impetus to the development of schemes which promote resource sharing and collaborative working between the statutory and voluntary sectors.

The Spirit in Mind strategy document (5) adopted by SWYFT in 2016 states 'The Spirit in Mind project recognises and seeks to draw upon the possibilities opened up by working with locally based faith and humanist organisations "spiritual partners" to significantly enhance the diversity and quality of support available to users of our service.' This is in line with recent government initiatives encouraging local government authorities to work in dialogue and partnership with the volunteering community and faith sectors to achieve better their service delivery and social action goals (6). This may include funding and commissioning, participation in governing bodies, committees and strategic partnerships.

Additional support for taking this initiative currently comes from the recently published NHS England Five Year Forward View for the development of services to 2021, which sees the contributions made by voluntary and social action as vital to achieving one of its prime goals of tackling financial shortfalls (7).

The Spirit in Mind project was launched at the Spirituality and Mental Health Conference at the University of Huddersfield in 2015. (8) In addition to the points mentioned earlier relating to government encouragement for partnership initiatives, the conference presentation included an overview of the current situation relating to faith organisations and community action.

Faith organisations remain integral to UK society and are at work in every community. A majority of the population self-identifies as having some kind of religious faith, spiritual beliefs or link to a religious tradition, though there is evidence that many church attendances are in decline (9). Nationally there are in excess of 11,000 accredited faith leaders (10), many of whom are involved in managing volunteers and paid staff, equipment and buildings. Faith organisations generally have strong local connections and a deep commitment to the well-being of their local communities. They also have a long track record of working with vulnerable people and have been at the forefront of many responses to contemporary social problems. The Spirit in Mind project recognises that faith organisations have a deep understanding of local needs and social priorities together with a strong motivation to support the flourishing of both their own membership and the wider community. In addition, faith groups and other spiritual organisations offer:

- A strong and well established volunteering ethos
- Physical resources often in central locations

- Direct channels into deprived neighbourhoods
- Good sources of local intelligence and knowledge
- A diversity of membership which crosses social and economic divides
- Strong national and international affiliations
- A record of being around for the long haul

Both locally and nationally there is no lack of evidence of faith-based social action demonstrating both diversity and innovation in response to identified needs. Recent examples include:

- Debt counselling
- Food banks
- Meditation for stress reduction
- Credit Unions
- Anti-racism and refugee work
- Street Angels (volunteers helping keep city centres safe at night by supporting vulnerable people)
- Homelessness projects (11)

Following the Spirit in Mind project's conference launch a number of locality-based workshops took place. Groups of 20 to 30 participants who had expressed interest in the project were invited to reflect on four key areas:

1. What is understood by 'spirituality' and what role does it have in promoting mental health and well-being? What sort of activities (with a spiritual focus) would you see as contributing to the promotion of mental health and well-being?
2. In relation to mental health support and promotion, what can faith organisations do that the statutory sector would find difficult or impossible?
3. What can faith organisations and the NHS do together that is more than either can do separately?

Workshop discussions confirmed a high level of community support and enthusiasm for taking the project to its next stage of development. This involved a business plan being drawn up detailing eligibility criteria for prospective partner organisations, including quality of organisational management and existing involvement in delivering spiritually vital programmes of activity.

The strategy document also requires prospective partner organisations to commit to a set of principles in accord with those developed by the All-Party Parliamentary Group on Faith and Society (12). These sought to address anxieties regarding possible proselytization by faith groups involved in social action. Partner organisations are required to commit to serving equally all local residents seeking to access the public services they offer without proselytization, irrespective of their religion, gender, marital status, race, ethnic origin, age, sexual orientation, mental capacity, long term condition or disability.

Now entering its next phase of development, Spirit in Mind has identified a number of front-runner pilot partner organisations and schemes. These include:

- A church and community centre to provide activities such as mindfulness-based meditation sessions to promote resilience and mental health.
- A Muslim community organisation to improve the understanding of mental health issues in the Muslim community and so improve access to services.
- A Christian organisation to develop bereavement counselling and support at a local level.
- A Methodist church to develop a programme of mental health awareness for its membership and the wider community.
- A Churches Together project working with asylum seekers and homeless people to up-skill its volunteers in understanding and responding to mental health issues.

At time of writing the initial pilots are being rolled out and evaluation and monitoring processes to track progress and outcomes are in the process of development.

The high level of interest in the project to date is indicative of recognition within wider society of the potential for improvement in the scale and diversity of services offered by models of collaborative working. The schemes currently under development put SWYFT in a strong position in leading the thinking in this area of development, which is of increasing interest to policy makers. In furthering SWYPT's key objective of providing services close to where people live and in championing innovative patterns of co-working and promoting a deeper understanding of the spiritual dimension to recovery and well-being, it also lends strong support to an emerging focus on compassion in health and social care.

A further positive outcome is the promotion of community cohesion provided by new models of collaborative working involving faith and religious groups. Most importantly, for service users and carers the project promises increased levels and choice of 'close to home' sources of support and a greater opportunity to engage with innovative approaches to promoting recovery from illness and the maintenance of well-being.

Case Study 2: Creative Minds

SWYFT introduced the Creative Minds strategy (13) in November 2011, and since then we've supported more than 250 creative projects in over 100 voluntary, third sector, not-for-profit organisations and other community groups to deliver creative, spiritual, sporting and environmentally based activities to more than 20,000 people. There was a general feeling in the organisation that the use of creative activities in health care settings can have a really huge impact on a person's well-being, by increasing their self-esteem so they feel confident to try new things, developing social skills as they meet new people, or providing a sense of purpose as they are actively engaged in meaningful activity that has a structure and aim. Where individuals have low expectations and poor self-image, the sense of achievement found in creativity gives them a chance to move away from negative or self-destructive patterns and habits and begin to write a new personal story that includes recovery.

Introducing the Creative Minds strategy was an opportunity for the Trust to build on its history of utilising creative approaches in partnership with local resources and facilities within local communities for local people. It also helped to raise awareness of the huge range of opportunities available for individuals to develop and grow creatively, with just a little support from the Trust and its partners. We have developed some excellent partnerships that are helping us to reach local people in a way that supports them to reach their recovery goals. We believe that we all have something inside us that responds to creativity – this may be through sport, dance, art, writing, walking, knitting, climbing, cycling, reading together and many other activities. Because we are all different and respond to different things, as an organisation, we need to make sure we can enable people to access a wide range of activities that appeal to diverse communities. Engaging in Creative Minds projects enables people to find passion and skills which help to restore hope, meaning and purpose in their lives – all recognised aspects of spirituality.

The main reason for developing the Creative Minds strategy was to meet a continued desire from service users and carers to be able to use more creative approaches to understand and support their health and well-being. This was a message that was constantly coming through our service user/carer dialogue groups and forums. Involving people is a strategic approach that has been a driving force in SWYFT. Putting people at the heart of the organisation, listening to and learning from people and working together to continually improve the quality of services. This approach, strongly embedded in our approach at Creative Minds, has driven our development. Our aim has been to build on and improve the systems that are already in place to support engagement, involvement, working together and to ensure people are more in control of their own health and well-being. Involving people and co-production helps us improve and develop approaches that respond positively and meaningfully to meet people's needs. Harnessing service user and carer knowledge and skills helps us to build better communities.

We held workshops across the communities the organisation serves that brought service users, carers, staff and community partners together to develop a strategy. A key part of the feedback stressed that engagement in creative activity helped people to challenge themselves constructively, imagine a different life for themselves and plan to move on to wider horizons away from the narrow confines and definitions of life as a receiver of health care. Creative engagement was also seen as an opportunity for people to engage as equals, to shift the power imbalance between care providers and the cared for, and for people to progress towards personal autonomy through developing a creative passion. The workshops helped to inform, develop and shape the Creative Minds strategy based on what creativity meant to individuals, the impact it had on their well-being and the type of activities they would like to be able to access. Another key finding was a need to ensure all the Trust's districts had equal opportunities for creative activity and learn from each other's good practice. Co-producing creative projects adds substantial value to the Trust's overall service offer by exploring areas beyond its current provision and also co-creating new and innovative solutions to the issues faced by individuals and communities (14). The approach builds and uses social capital to create and restore a community spirit that enables people to reach their potential and live well in their communities in keeping with the Trust's mission. It also helps to challenge the stigma and isolation people with mental health issues can experience.

We wanted to bring Creative Minds to life and be much more than a black-and-white document that sits on a shelf that nobody sees. We wanted a strong image for Creative Minds and we developed a colourful logo and produced the strategy in a magazine format (15) to get into community venues, grabbing people's attention. Our website (16) promotes what we do, providing links to our partners. We organised live events in mainstream venues such as art galleries and theatres to showcase the talents of people who use our services and challenge stigma. We have also developed a suite of films featuring participants telling their stories and promoting the benefits linked to social media channels (2).

A key component of the popularity of Creative Minds was to define creativity in the broadest sense to take into account not only the contribution of the arts, but also the contribution sports and other recreational and leisure activities can make to improved health and well-being. This has given participants greater choice that includes not only music, dance, poetry but also football, walking, gardening and knitting. Creative Minds is altering perceptions of what mental health is about. Creative approaches offer a different way of engaging with communities and have worked particularly well with people who have traditionally been more difficult to engage.

A major aim of Creative Minds was to build a strong infrastructure of community and voluntary organisations able to work with the Trust providing excellent creative projects for all who access our services. Therefore, partnerships and co-production were core to the conception and development of Creative Minds. It not only shows our commitment as an organisation to having a creative approach to service delivery but also showcases our passion for working in partnership with our communities. Creative Minds has provided a way to not only build on existing good practice in our services, but also to work more closely with a wide range of community organisations enhancing our service provision by delivering innovative, transformative and meaningful health and well-being projects. We have a network of internal and external champions whose passion and commitment to creative approaches has helped to bring Creative Minds to life. We are now using this infrastructure to help embed this different way of working in all that we do.

This partnership approach was built on an earlier project developed by the Trust called Inspire. This was essentially an artist in residence scheme which enabled practitioners from various disciplines such as photography, painting and music to run creative workshops in the Trust. Partners from this work were approaching us with requests to match community funding for further projects, but the Trust was not able to respond in the timescales dictated by funders. In response to this issue we developed our Creative Partners programs within Creative Minds. This provides a fund for matching community funding and setting up our partners as preferred suppliers. For every pound the Trust invests it gets at least a pound match from community sources such as Big Lottery, Arts Council, Lankelly Chase and others. On top of this, most of our partners have a large body of volunteers supporting them and this adds further resources and social value and often provides opportunities for those using Trust services to contribute to something meaningful.

Where we have invested funding into creative projects we have encouraged partners to find cash-matched funding or in-kind contributions such as volunteer time, and in the majority of cases this has been successful and often exceeded expectations. Matched funding enables us to increase the size and scope of the project and increases the number of people who benefit. This initially proved difficult to facilitate due to organisational red tape but it has become easier by encouraging community organisations and groups to become formal Creative Partners in advance of any decision making. Matched funding has come from different sources including statutory organisations, local authorities and clinical commissioning groups. Our partnership approach has provided the governance those funders need to invest confidently in smaller community organisations, with the reputation and size of our organisation providing the necessary reassurances.

Creative Minds has provided an infrastructure and a framework enabling creative community partnerships to flourish across the Trust's communities in Barnsley, Calderdale, Kirklees and Wakefield. They have harnessed a shared passion for the arts, sports, crafts and leisure activities and a belief that creativity should be at the heart of recovery-focused services. We believe that this approach has promoted the inclusion of people who use our services into the wider community. It has strengthened the belief that creative approaches improve the quality of people's lives in the present and in the future by acting as building blocks for better self-generated health outcomes. We are now starting to see how this work is impacting on our working practices in a variety of ways, and in a significant way how it impacts on the lives of people.

The principles and philosophy of Creative Minds seemed to strike a chord with many people. We have initiated a genuine social movement of which people want to be part, and for which people feel a sense of ownership. The general definition of a social movement (17) is collective action by individuals who have voluntarily come together around a common cause; they often involve radical action which may conflict with accepted norms and ways of doing things. This seems to resonate with people involved in Creative Minds and fitted with theories being developed at the NHS Institute for Innovation and Improvement.

> The social movements perspective fundamentally challenges the ways that we have learnt to organise and lead change in the NHS. It advocates that health care improvement strategies need to extend beyond the top down programme by programme approach to embrace a concept of citizen led (health care staff and/or user) change that draws upon unstructured and largely self-organising autocatalytic (self-fuelling) factors. Given the NHS Improvement Plan themes of grass roots engagement in health improvement and individual and community empowerment, perhaps this is a set of ideas whose time has come (18).
>
> (Helen Bevan NHS institute for Innovation and Improvement, 2009.)

One of the key factors in the success of our approach has been shared leadership and co-production. Working together with everyone having a say has been quite crucial when working with people who are feeling marginalised and ignored. We have been very lucky to be working in such a values-driven organisation where everyone is appreciated for their contribution. Having a chief executive who is an artist and a director of finance who sings in a choir means that these staff members fully understand the benefits and fully support this approach. This has meant that barriers were removed and replaced with a solution-focussed culture that enabled the approach to develop.

We have a governance group that helped us develop a framework for turning the ideas for Creative Minds into practical approaches and projects. The group provides assurance and guidance on the business/financial elements and ensures Creative Minds plays an influential role in organisational development and service transformation. The governance group is chaired by the Trust's chief executive and includes other executives and non-executive directors, service users/carers and representatives from our partner organisations. The group also guides the strategic direction of Creative Minds, enabling the free flow of ideas to ensure the approach stays fresh and innovative. Because the Trust covers a large geographic area, we have a network of local collectives which make decisions about local projects and developments. These are made up of service users/carers, staff and community representatives. All partners are approved through the Trust procurement process to ensure they meet our governance standards. We have a scaled-down process for service user–led projects.

Creative Minds enables us to work in a different way for the combined benefit of people who use our services, their carers, our staff and our local communities. Our plans have a recovery focus, with people retaining control over their own health and well-being; Creative Minds helps us to do this. SWYFT is in a unique position due to our strong foundation of harnessing creative potential through the development of Creative Minds. This has already initiated a change in culture whereby our staff consider all aspects of people's lives and doesn't just focus on delivering specific treatments. The approach builds and uses social capital to create and restore a community spirit that enables people to reach their potential and live well in their communities.

Evaluation

We have done lot of work to evaluate the impact that Creative Minds is having. Personal accounts from those who have taken part in projects and the positive impact it has had on their lives have been captured through case studies.

All Creative Minds projects carry out their own evaluations, which demonstrate the positive impact of the projects. Using a variety of health improvement tools has made it hard to draw broader conclusions. We have recently developed a shortened version of the Warwick & Edinburgh Mental Well-being Scale evaluation tool (19). All projects will use this in the future, ensuring that we have a consistent approach to evaluation that generates results which can be used to draw wider conclusions.

We are also working with the University of Huddersfield health research team to develop a full university-led approach using participatory research methods (20). This will give us a richer picture of the improvements over a longer time period.

The impact that Creative Minds is having on the recovery of people is evident in the stories they tell.

Diane's Story

Never in my life have I done art; I just thought I'd give it a go. I went along and I absolutely loved it. I think the main thing for me is the confidence that it's given me. I'm a totally different person to the one that walked through the door.

I was a quivering, shivering wreck on 21 tablets a day – and 20 months later I've been off medication for nine months and my children are amazed that one person can change so much in such a short space of time. They never thought it would be possible and I didn't either – but it is.

Without Creative Minds I would not be here today.

Having been in and out of mental health services for 20+ years, I found myself involved with them again due to many external factors. The service was, to say the least, disgusting. I was not treated as a person or with respect for my views on my own care. I would like to say that I think this is a one off, but sadly I know of several people who have received the same treatment.

By chance, at the end of 2011, whilst waiting for a psychological assessment, I noticed a note about art for wellbeing. Having never drawn and never had the ability to draw, what drew me to the note I will never know. I rang the number and spoke to a very nice reassuring voice telling me that I could attend the next session starting beginning of December.

I arrived and did the taster sessions and loved it. I actually drew a teasel. (I had to redraw it at home again as my daughters did not believe that I had drawn it!!) I was hooked. I continued to go and each week I felt more confident and was actually excited at going to 'art'. Instead of taking sleeping tablets, I got my art pad out and sketched when things were on my mind. I was sleeping like I had never slept before. I began to feel 'reasonable' and 'well'.

I attended the first paid sessions and then again with the second half funded sessions. Luckily for the next sessions one of the other students (who had seen my confidence and health improve) was willing to sponsor me for another round of sessions. I was totally hooked at this point and was now trying my hand at painting. I have become part of the furniture at artworks (whether they like it or not!).

When I asked my psychiatrist for some support I was refused (I was on the waiting list for psychological services so my consultant said that was the only help I needed even though the waiting list was over 18 months long). I had nothing but the support of the Creative Minds and the wonderful tutors at Artworks to keep me going through a very tough time in my life. Without them I have no doubt that I would not be here today to thank you for helping and getting involved in Creative Minds.

I have sold a couple of my works of art!! I attend any meetings I can regarding mental health/ Creative Minds to improve the service (or in creative minds case to tell as many people as I can about how wonderful it is). I am medication free (after 20+years) and doing really well. I finally feel free of the fog that has blighted my life for so many years. My daughters can all see the difference in me and are so pleased they finally have a mum that isn't so depressed that I cannot get out of bed or cope with everyday life let alone all the issues that arise within it.

I am under no illusion that I have bipolar and depressive disorder and that I will have this for the rest of my life. I also know that I can focus my 'fog' on my drawing/painting. Life is not always easy and there are always issues and problems arising within it, but I feel I have an outlet and a way of expressing that pain without it being such a huge part of my life that I cannot cope. I feel, for the first time I can ever remember, alive. I want to wake up each day. I want to go out and see beautiful things that I can draw/paint. Most importantly I want to live.

Being a part of Creative Minds and attending Art sessions, my daughters have a mum and I have a life.

Realising the Value

In 2016 Creative Minds was selected to be a local partner site for NHS England's Realising the Value Programme (21), part of the NHS Five Year Forward View (7) supported by a consortium led by Nesta (formerly National Endowment for Science, Technology and the Arts), an independent charity that works to increase the innovation capacity of the UK. The programme seeks to enable the health and care system to support people to have the knowledge, skills and confidence to play an active role in managing their own health and care and to work with communities and their assets. The aims of this approach fitted very well with Creative Minds. We feel a fully integrated partnership approach to developing group activities is an important element to improving the health and well-being of people in secondary health care services.

In our experience there is a strong NHS culture that drives the way individuals and communities approach and manage their health and well-being. This is often underpinned by a 'medical model' that is managed and controlled by doctors and nurses who are perceived as the experts. The 'doctor/nurse know best' approach was dominant in previous generations and still has some resonance today. There is a general move towards shifting the power balance away from a health system controlled by experts to one that is much more in the hands of the individual/community. In mental health services this shift has a long history based on a service user empowerment model and an anti-psychiatry movement. If we are to enable the health and care system to support people to have the knowledge, skills and confidence to play an active role in managing their own health and care we have to facilitate a shift to a more socially-/community-driven recovery model. Empowerment of individuals to take more ownership of their health and well-being is the direction of travel with more coproduction and service user–led activities.

Fully understanding this context is critical to ensuring that people have the right guidance and support to make the right steps on their journey of recovery and why we feel a fully integrated partnership approach is the right path. In terms of our approach at SWYFT, a strong driver was the development of our mission to help people to reach their potential and live well in their community, already discussed, which moves us away from symptom management and towards a more community-oriented approach. At Creative Minds we have built and developed on this foundation, based on strong community partnerships that link in a complementary way to secondary mental health care services.

One of the key factors in developing strong partnerships is decisions about how project funding and development are made. Our bids for project funding are assessed by the Creative Minds team and locality collective, made up of service users/carers and trust staff. We use the following categories to assess the suitability of new project proposals:

1. Does the project fit with the Creative Minds Strategy and organisation's mission?
2. Does the project demonstrate projected health, well-being and other benefits?
3. How will the project be implemented including links into Trust Services?
4. How does the project demonstrate cost-effectiveness, including matched funding? (22)

The collectives are also looking for a balanced portfolio of projects across the Trust districts, taking into account the types of activity, the client group and the service that will benefit. Where projects show a weakness in any of the categories, we try to work with the organisation to look for a way forward.

Some of the Benefits

Recovery: Many participants have told us that getting involved with one of the creative activities has made a difference to their own well-being as well as helping them feel as though they are a part of a community.

Prevention: Creative approaches can help engage with people in communities with the highest levels of deprivation and hardship. Creative programmes have been shown to promote better health and well-being in vulnerable individuals and foster social integration, community strength and cohesion.

Reducing stigma: Showcasing positive artistic achievement challenges negative stereotypes and celebrates participants' talents and abilities, conferring value and esteem in the process. Spending time together in mutually valued activities over long periods of time improves community attitudes and acceptance of people with mental health problems.

Early intervention: Early engagement with 'softer' techniques avoids deterioration of health needs and the need for more expensive and intrusive interventions.

Personalised care: Services need to develop the capacity to offer real choice to individuals to purchase self-determined packages of care. Access to creative activities is popular with service users, and therefore likely to be an important component of the new market of social care.

Multi-agency commissioning: The creativity agenda offers real opportunities for partnerships with other creative groups and agencies, in the process increasing the range of creative resources and approaches available to service users.

Innovation: As well as supporting service users to seek creative and imaginative approaches to support their personal growth and development, the creativity agenda can be used at all levels within the organisation to seek innovative approaches to client care, team development, service development and organisational management.

Value for money: Providing creative activity is often more cost effective than many other medical or therapeutic interventions. There are opportunities to lever additional funds through partnerships working with external arts/health agencies.

Strengthening transition: Working with creative agencies in the community builds links to a range of new opportunities in the wider community, supporting progress away from acute services towards greater autonomy and independence.

Resilience – individual and community: Creative approaches have been shown to be effective in building cohesion and strength in vulnerable communities and providing significant gains in personal resilience and recovery from mental and physical ill health.

Conclusion

Spirit in Mind and Creative Minds provide an infrastructure and framework enabling a more holistic person-centred approaches to grow and develop. They have also enabled community partnerships to flourish across the Trust's area and empowered individuals to have a real stake in future developments. We feel we have harnessed a shared passion and a belief that spirituality and creativity should be at the heart of recovery-focused services. This approach is now embraced by SWYFT and is seen as a major enhancement of the Trusts service offer. We also recognise that these approaches will not suit everyone; a broad level of choice and the opportunity to respond to unmet need where there are gaps are offered. These approaches work in synergy with more traditional medical, nursing, psychological and social approaches to mental health care. Developing these approaches as part of organisational strategy and delivered as part of a fully integrated approach with full engagement of Trust staff and people who use Trust services has also enabled them to become part of the organisations culture. All decisions are co-produced with representatives from service users, carers and Trust staff to ensure that the projects are more likely to meet people's needs and they are supported by services. Although these programs will not meet everyone's needs, they remain broad enough to offer a large selection of choices for individuals. Spirit in Mind and Creative Minds are reconfiguring the future of the Trust's services, changing the benchmarks through arts, sports, recreation and partnerships with community and faith organisations. They are developing effective, inexpensive, non-pharmacological locally configured services to supplement and sometimes replace more traditional models of provision. The end result is a powerful redefinition of what constitutes good mental health services. The programs encourage service users and practitioners to engage for mutual benefit, provide an opportunity for people to engage as equals, and shift the imbalance between providers and participants. We agree with Paul Crawford that:

> There is an urgent need for compassionate design of health care services. The recent Francis Report in the UK highlights that the systems and cultures of care in some of our hospitals need to be overhauled. Quite aside from enhancing the management of health care services or revisiting professional standards, it would be timely to consider how the arts and humanities can help to create more friendly, warm and homely environments for patients and practitioners alike and soften the 'production-line' mentality and target-obsessed culture of modern health care (23).

Through Spirit in Mind and Creative Minds, our staff play football in the same team, sing in the same choir, paint in the same art session and practice mindfulness with people who use Trust services.

References

1. NHS Foundation Trust. Health and Social Care (Community Health And Standards) Act 2003. Chapter 43, NHS Foundation Trusts; 2003, p 1.
2. Creative Minds. Films. Available at: southwestyorkshire.nhs.uk/quality-innovation/creative-minds/creative-minds-films (accessed 9/9/16).
3. Equality Act 2010. Chapter 1, section 10. Available at: gov.uk/discrimination-your-rights/types-of-discrimination (accessed 15/9/16).
4. Mayo M, Blake G, Diamond J, Foot J, Gidley B, Shukra K, Yamit M. Community empowerment and community cohesion: parallel agendas for community building in England? The Centre on Migration, Policy, and Society (COMPAS). 2009. Available at: compas.ox.ac.uk/2009/gidley-etal_jsi_2009/ (accessed 9/9/16).
5. Gartland M. Spirit in Mind Strategy. SWYFT. 2016. Available at: southwestyorkshire.nhs.uk/your-wellbeing/spirit-in-mind/ (accessed 9/9/16).
6. Birdwell J. Commissioning faith groups to provide services that can save money and strengthen a community. Faithful Providers. Demos. 2012. Available at: demos.co.uk/files/Faithful_Providers_-_web.pdf?1358533399 (accessed 8/16).
7. NHS England. Five year forward view, 23 October 2014. Available at: england.nhs.uk/wp-content/uploads/2014/10/5yfv-web.pdf (accessed 8/16).

8. University of Huddersfield/SWYFT. Spirituality and Mental Health Conference. 2015. Available at: hud.ac.uk/news/2015/may/spiritualityandmentalhealthconference.php (accessed 8/16).

9. Brown A. Faith no more: how the British are losing their religion. *The Guardian*. 2015. Available at: theguardian.com/commentisfree/belief/2015/apr/14/british-christianity-trouble-religion-comeback (accessed 8/16).

10. Department for Communities and Local Government. *Faith Communities and Pandemic Flu, Guidance for Faith Communities and Local Influenza Pandemic Committees*. London: Department for Communities and Local Government; 2009, p 5.

11. Joseph Rowntree Foundation. *Faith in Urban Regeneration? Engaging Faith Communities in Urban Regeneration*. York: Joseph Rowntree Foundation; 2003.

12. All Party Parliamentary Group on Faith and Society. Summary Report. 2013. Available at: faithaction.net/wp-content/uploads/2014/12/APPG_Report_2013.pdf (accessed 9/9/16).

13. SWYFT. Creative Minds Strategy. 2011. (Due for revision December 2016). Available at: southwestyorkshire.nhs.uk/quality-innovation/creative-minds/our-strategy (accessed 8/16).

14. Realpe A, Wallace LM. What is co-production? The Health Foundation. 2010. Available at: personcentredcare.health.org.uk/sites/default/files/resources/what_is_co-production.pdf (accessed 8/16).

15. SWYFT. Creative Minds Magazine. 2011. Available at: southwestyorkshire.nhs.uk/quality-innovation/creative-minds/magazine (accessed 8/16).

16. SWYFT. Creative Minds. Available at: southwestyorkshire.nhs.uk/quality-innovation/creative-minds (accessed 8/16).

17. Melucci A. The new social movements a theoretical approach. *Social Science Information*. 1980; 19(2): 199–226.

18. Bevan H. Social movement thinking: a set of ideas whose time has come? 2009. Available at: webarchive.nationalarchives.gov.uk/20081113000758/http://www.institute.nhs.uk/quality_and_value/introduction/helen_bevan_on_social_movement_thinking%3a_a_set_of_ideas_whose_time_has_come%3f.html (accessed 9/9/16).

19. NHS Health Scotland. Measuring mental wellbeing. 2015. Available at: healthscotland.com/scotlands-health/population/Measuring-positive-mental-health.aspx (accessed 8/16)

20. Bergold J, Thomas S. Participatory research methods: a methodological approach in motion. *Forum: Qualitative Social Research*. 2012; 13(1):Art. 30. Available at: qualitative-research.net/index.php/fqs/article/view/1801/3334 (accessed 9/9/16).

21. The Health Foundation/Nesta. At the heart of health: realising the value of people and communities. 2016. Available at: nesta.org.uk/sites/default/files/at_the_heart_of_health_-_realising_the_value_of_people_and_communities.pdf (accessed 8/16).

22. Walters, P. 2016. Creative Minds Strategic Lead March 2016. Available at: southwestyorkshire.nhs.uk/wp-content/uploads/2014/07/Creative-Minds-Project-Application-Form-Guidance-for-constituted-groups-2016-17.doc (accessed 9/9/16).

23. Crawford P. Urgent need for compassionate design of healthcare services. 2013. Available at: healthhumanities.org/blog/view/0/12 (accessed 9/9/16).

Using Social Role Valorisation to Make Services Sensitive to Spiritual Need

12

Kevin Bond

Background

What does average look like? Not necessarily a question you would want to be asked in relation to treatment and caring services for vulnerable people, but nevertheless a question asked by an accountable clinical lead officer in a Clinical Commissioning Group (CCG) responsible for commissioning health care services. Why would somebody ask such a question – don't we strive for excellence anymore? Perhaps in times of financial restraint vulnerable groups always come off worse (1).

In this chapter I examine the problems, the lack of understanding, the 'make do', 'good enough' attitude, or at worst, discrimination, that pervade services for people from vulnerable groups. Ideas are presented on how we can help people who are undervalued by society in general get a better sense of their own worth and value as part of their total experience in mental health services. This ties in with the concept of spirituality as what gives people is a sense of meaning and purpose; indeed it is a treatment of sorts in itself.

So what is actually going on here? Are these attitudes symptomatic of a time in which targets and metrics have finally eclipsed the intangibles of the soul and the spirit and their importance to the final outcomes in care and treatment for people? It is no doubt true that 'intellectualising' issues, as described in the psychological literature over many decades (2), can remove something of the emotion that should accompany them. It is sometimes used in the NHS as a defence mechanism, to avoid the pain we might feel in empathising with stories of individual suffering. We do this by removing the sense of the individual person and failing to realise that we too could find ourselves in the same situation. We hear of stigma (3) and the need for educating the public on issues such as mental health, but this is a matter for those commissioning and working within health services as well as the public (4), as we also often discriminate and stigmatise. I often hear disparaging terms such as 'frequent flyer' used to describe people who use accident and emergency departments a lot, or other services. Many of the people so identified are vulnerable and cannot achieve the care they require in other ways. Sometimes the very professionals who give these labels are the ones who fail to provide more accessible and appropriate services. We know that people with long-term mental health problems are likely to die between 15 and 20 years younger than the rest of us (5), largely due to lifestyle, preventable physical illness and disparity of access to physical health tests and services.

Social Role Valorisation

Not much of an opening about the importance of 'spirituality' (6) and its applicability in terms of competent practice (7,8); but bear with me, as this knowledge of the tendency to devalue marginalised groups is crucial in the design of effective services that enhance people's spiritual well-being and sense of self. In 2016, the King's Fund (9) reported that 40% Mental Health Trusts had seen their income fall over the previous two years. This was on top of a decrease in income reported by 45% of Mental Health Trusts in the previous year and despite promises in plans from nearly 90% of Care Commissioning Groups (CCGs) that funding would increase in 2015-16. This also happened despite Government promises and the Royal College of Psychiatrists campaign for parity of esteem (10). Hardly a day goes by without discussion of poor resourcing of mental health. Eating disorders, young people and new parents have been the focus of attention most recently. This clash between priorities and funding is not very uplifting for the soul! However, this dissonance between stated priorities and spending exposes the devaluing of marginalised groups as part of the problem. Understanding this helps us understand how to fix it.

The way other people treat them is possibly even more important to how people with mental health problems feel and to their life outcomes than their psychiatric diagnosis (11,12). So what exactly is this theory of social role valorisation (SRV) and how does it help?

It's relatively simple, but such a clever theory that the author believes it has not dated one bit, despite all the more recent anti-stigma work and all the acknowledgement of the concept as a key problem in outcomes. The theory of SRV was described by Wolf Wolfensberger in 1983 (13) and developed from his earlier concept of 'normalization' (14,15). He developed his ideas in the context of how people with learning disabilities might be treated and what might help them to be better integrated and accepted in society. The author of this chapter was working on elements of the closure and re-provision of a big mental hospital at the time and it changed the way he has thought about the issues involved completely. Every service that he has ever run, every design ever done or suggested, has always been underpinned by a simple idea: SRV.

Wolfensberger wrote about it at length, but the essence of SRV is that people with long-term illnesses or disabilities are already devalued by society. This causes them a great disadvantage in terms of other people's expectations of them. There are implicit questions about how they will behave, what they will achieve and whether they are reliable, or safe to be around. In a sheltered environment, we can treat them, 'fix' them and help them develop a sense of confidence. However, when they seek to re-engage with the wider world, if nothing has changed about the way they are viewed and treated by others, then progress will swiftly be eroded and relapse may ensue. Unless we help to find people 'valued roles' (16) more damage will be done. According to Osburn (17), Wolfensberger went so far as to say that society was happy to have some people removed, kept away, disadvantaged, or even wished them destroyed. If we consider the treatment of people with mental health problems over time, we can see the truth in this at many levels. One does not have to go too far in mental health services to find some 'old timer' (like the author) talking about the ills of the big, old mental hospitals and negative effects they had on people. Of course, there were some positives too, and you will still find staff who talk about the big mental hospitals still with conflicting affection. What is true is that 'we' as a society have often been prepared to do things to people with mental health problems that we would not wish done to us. At best we might consider these necessary or understandable, at worst that people with mental health problems simply have less value.

Goffman's 1961 (18) analysis of 'total institutions' and the damage they did to people's individuality and their 'souls' was also influential. He drew clear parallels between all total institutions. (Restrictive and very orderly institutions which affect all levels of functioning and choice of those people who are members of them, or indeed confined in them. Prisons, mental health institutions and military bases are examples, because almost all of the activities of people within them are managed and overseen by others.) Didn't we fix all that by closing the mental hospitals? Certainly there are not as many large institutions as there used to be. We have a different set of standards now, don't we? But do we really, or did we simply curb the most obvious ethical failings, where treatment may be given, but care and stewardship of the spirit is still, at times, so poor? We have, for instance, for many years as a society felt it wrong in some way to put children who require a 'home' in large institutions of 30, 40, 50 even 100, yet we seem happy to do this to older people, particularly those who have confusion or dementia, and to add to this we have the misnomer of care 'home', or 'nursing home' as a title. Do they conform to any of the criteria we might expect of a home, which might be defined by control over one's environment, choice and privacy? We know standards are additionally often very poor, yet somehow it is understandable, not affordable to do otherwise in the 'social care' environment of today. Some have postulated these are the total institutions of today (19). We have, though, invented a new language for this: terms such as 'failings in the care pathway', which remove the personal nature of the abuse. These and the new somewhat smaller hospitals (but worryingly getting larger again in the urge to do things 'at scale', that pervades the NHS), are the new institutions and, without great care in design and day-to-day running, they still do great damage to individuality, to the spirit, to the soul, even to the 'outcome' in today's language. So that, whilst they might offer up-to-date treatment, by not offering great care, they may not offer all that needs to be present to gain great outcomes. The environments might be prettier colours and provide individual rooms for patients, but the need goes so much deeper than that. In our modern designs and modelling, we still often do the damage and 'harms' that were described by Wolfensberger years ago. We still devalue people with persistent illness and fail to offer them the support they need.

A recent example, on a unit for older people with confusion due to physical illness, highlights this well. At a point when her physical illness deteriorated, a woman was moved four times to different wards around the general hospital. Whilst this was, of course, genuinely aimed at curing her illness, clearly it had other wider effects on her overall care and increased her disorientation and bewilderment. When these concerns were raised, a consultant rightly argued the treatment had worked, her illness was 'better'. This was true, but it was equally true that we had somehow damaged other parts of her and she was not restored to her former wholeness. It could be said that her 'spirit was broken'. The final outcome was not as good as it could have been and she was unable to return to her own home. Many examples of the inadequacies of hospital environments and their models of care for older people with complex needs can be cited. This is epitomised in the Mid-Staffordshire Hospitals Inquiry (Francis Report) (19). In the absence of real alternatives, we keep sending confused people into general hospitals not adapted to meet their human needs in a holistic way. We do this even though we know outcomes are likely to be poor. We have nowhere else to send them, and the NHS, in its present organisational form, seems incapable of finding effective alternatives. Nobody seems to be able to get fundamental change with any ease, despite the public outcry that followed the Francis Report. There have been some changes to training, and some slightly more friendly environments have been provided. However there has not been a really systematic understanding of the damage done and the full 'cure' required.

Us and Them

The truth is we all are wired to assess quickly who is 'us' and who is 'them'. We have known about stereotyping (21) and labelling theory, as first described in 1928 (22), for a long time. We know that we need to fight against the urge to make such cursory judgements on people. Yet we still do separate 'us' and 'them' and it is possible to do things to 'them', that we cannot feel justified in doing to 'us'. This is the root of most 'isms' and as a society we feel that mental health 'patients' are somehow less valuable, less worthy and hence need less facilities. Are they not perhaps dangerous? Unpredictable? Unreliable? One in four people will suffer mental health problems in their lifetime (23) but who really wants to believe it might happen to them? Perhaps it is better to try to ignore it? Providers of mental health services themselves are not always much better. Our facilities are often poorly designed for human interaction, with overemphasis on security and sometimes shabby and devaluing, damaged and broken. Is this the best we feel we can do in the circumstances? Or maybe we, too, buy into some of the labelling that associates itself so quickly with 'schizophrenic', 'demented' or 'depressive'? Or have we just become desensitised? Treat a person constantly as potentially dangerous and they will be dangerous, as unreliable and they may become so, as unable to make their own choices and of little value and we will inevitably crush something of their soul.

Perhaps there should be our own application in mental health of *primum non nocere* (first do no harm; 24). This principle applies to all people requiring help, who being ill, are devalued and disempowered in some ways. The people who come to us in mental health services may already feel very exposed and potentially find it demeaning to come for help. They may feel traumatised to have to seek help and shame that they are not coping. They have to bare all to us; to allow us into their very souls.

First do no harm, do not do anything that makes them feel less equal, less important, less worthy. Concentrating in everything we do to avoid adding to that damage, concentrating on healing the spirit (7), not just treating the illness, should be the stuff of all good mental health care.

So the 'cure' is to get people 'valued roles' in tandem with their treatment; all that we do must offer value. First do no more harm. The problem though, is that experience suggests it is quite a complex and subtle business. The way staff behave, how aware they are, the total environment, how treatment is offered and given, the way we dress, the opportunities people are presented with or not, the way people are addressed and many more things all influence how people feel and their sense of self. Worse still, from a perspective of addressing the issues, small things can often change things so much and this requires real attention to detail. A single notice on the wall in an otherwise excellent environment can set an 'institutional' tone. One single overly clinical item in a home can immediately remove all the other feeling of homeliness. In addition, all people need to be treated as individuals and whilst common ground is present, there are also areas in which one person might take offense and another not. The idea of a *therapeutic milieu* is still being refined in mental health (25) and for wider purposes as well (26). It is a devilishly difficult thing to define and engineer. However, the principle of offering value and making our services good enough for our own friends and family is our standard for our design of models of care and treatment and the environments in which we provide this. So we need to understand that the people we see are disadvantaged, are often damaged or at risk of damage way beyond that caused by any illness. They are often seen by society in general, and sometimes even by ourselves, as having less value than those who are 'well'. These attitudes and the behaviours they cause can inadvertently do people further harm. Recognising these prejudices in ourselves and others is the key to dealing with them and providing services that truly value the people we serve.

Designing and Providing New Models of Service

This kind of thinking is vital in designing new services and models, and in the author's view fits well alongside more recent 'recovery'-oriented ideation widely cited and explored from the 1990s in mental health literature (27). Clearly, involving staff and people who use services in design is important, but without posing the right questions and setting the background to what we are trying to achieve, we are unlikely to address all the needs. At a time of great change, staff may externalise their own insecurities and concentrate on areas such as physical security, safety and clinical efficacy. Subtleties like the overall milieu and the need to support the sense of meaning, purpose and personal value that people using our services need may be neglected. People who use services will also often struggle to see beyond their experiences in the past to a truly new approach. In addition to this, in the NHS it is often easier and safer to copy what has already been done, even if that is flawed. Innovation is more likely to provoke blame. It is easier to repeat than develop. This is bit of a minefield then, so what things may help?

Key Concepts

1. People who use and work in services need some influence in those services, both in their design and operation. They need to have some real power against a framework that helps them to evaluate the issues. Care needs to be a partnership between people who use services and the people who staff them. A real partnership is essential; simple consultation (we listen but do not act) is not enough. Note I say 'people' throughout.
2. Services, particularly those where residential staff or admission is required, need to be on a more domestic scale. This will help in providing truly facilitative services, not creating dependency and keeping people functioning to a level they can cope with safely. It will also be easier to create a more human feel.

3. Training. Really working with all staff to help them understand their power and influence for good or bad and the subtleties at play. Asking staff to view services as if they were using them, and becoming aware of what might offend or cause problems. Asking them to visualise their loved ones receiving the services.

4. Organisational design. Making sure the whole system relates to and meets the needs of people who use it. No 'back office' staff that do not know or meet those people who use services. Training 'non-clinical' staff to understand core concepts, having no managers who are not engaged with people who use services. Everyone in services knowing what services are there to do.

5. Language. Use the word 'people' a lot. Long-winded perhaps, but reminds us all that is what we do, 'work with people'. Spring-clean all ugly, disempowering language, jargon or 'ies', 'ics' and 'ers' (self-harmers, frequent flyers, junkies, attention seekers, schizophrenics etc.). Really spring clean all the rubbish we talk as code to identify our club; if it can't be understood by the public, either explain it or don't use it. Educate people who use services to expect to understand and to ask, and feel OK to do so. Oh yes, and stop all the NHS weird management-speak like the constant urge to say 'big beasts' and 'working in silos'. Let's stop 'talking in silos' – I am very proud of that one, I coined it and you can use it at your next management meeting – 'let's all stop talking in silos'.

6. Training. Yes, more training; but this time using people who know: the people who use the services! Try to have people who use services involved in all training and where appropriate be trained in things together too. Share the knowledge that makes you an 'expert'; don't hold it because it makes you feel special. Give it to others, then find more.

7. Blunt the clinical and security features. Just because a place is registered a hospital, it does not have to look like it. Although security features may be required, if you do not want negative effects in terms of labelling, then make these as subtle and unobtrusive as possible. Such features are disempowering if not carefully dealt with. They shout loudly of a lack of trust.

8. Make the maximum amount of the space available accessible to the public and those using facilities. Reduce 'staff only' areas. If the facilities aren't relaxing enough for everyone, make then make them so; if they are not clean enough for everyone, then make them so, and if staff are not comfortable amongst those they serve, then train them to be so.

9. Invite the public in. Have public schemes, sports teams, open clubs, work on the press and media about their portrayal of mental health. Answer their questions, demystify.

10. Create 'valued roles' for people. Let staff see peoples' talents as well as the public. Try to run services with the people who use them and use your facilities and their needs as training and employment schemes. This helps not just the public see people differently, but us too. Someone who wants help can move from being a vulnerable recipient, when you have eaten a good meal cooked by them, to a chef who has a mental health problem.

Easy then? Maybe not, but start with questioning all. A wise old mental health chief executive (not quite so old as he should be for this wisdom perhaps!) said to me once something along the lines of 'but Kevin we were trained to know what we did was wrong'. Maybe the one advantage of the institution was that at least we knew change had to come, but at best we were told to go ahead and change the world. It was our duty to try to really make a difference to the lives our system had damaged. We were proud of that when we got it right. There could and should be a brave new world. Have we (the generation that experienced that), passed on some of that urge to redress, that knowledge that what we do is wrong and can be improved?

So having posed so many questions, raised so many issues, questioned the core of what we do, what then has practically worked to the author's knowledge, what can be done for real?

Some Real-Life Examples

In the following paragraphs I offer a few examples of things I think really made a difference. From a service failing by any measure, to NAViGO social enterprise, one that is far better rated by those who use it and staff it. One that achieves in large measure much better outcomes, but better still, seems to truly facilitate healthier, more equal relationships between people who staff it and people who use it, and has many bespoke features. Many people who use the service refer to staff and themselves as 'we' and where their needs are cyclic often volunteer, or maintain contact in between real difficulties to maintain stability. This is a service where informal contacts are allowed and encouraged, so that people can receive reassurance, a sense of community and stay involved with us to ensure that when they need it, they can get help they want and trust. Where, in between any necessary episodes of formal care, a person might simply have lunch in one of our public cafes to achieve some reassurance with a manager, nurse or therapist. Or they may just keep in touch with an occasional email, maybe by calling in for a coffee.

NAViGO

Firstly, the organisation itself endeavours to gain more equal relationships between people, ensuring that everything is designed to help people be seen as individuals, but also to give people influence. It is designed with the purest sense of what might be described as co-production in approaches to involving people with their services (28). NAViGO is a bespoke social enterprise, so some of the detailed activities and designs may not be directly transferable, but could be remodelled to fit other organisations. NAViGO (the name is simply an amalgam of navigating, going forward, a tip of the hat to North East Lincolnshire's nautical links) has, for instance, a voting membership of staff, people who use services, carers and genuinely interested local people. They all have equal voting rights – yes, equal voting rights – and on things that matter too! The CEO's appointment requires periodic re-approval. The organisation's chair and membership representatives are elected as full non-executive directors on the board. If a surplus is made by working more efficiently, or by schemes that are run in excess of the standard contract, large grant schemes (£100,000) are both designed/suggested and voted on by the membership. More than this though, it is in the fabric of the organisation that wisdom is achieved by doing things together. People who use services are involved in everything, all the meetings, all the interviews, most training and just being wherever they wish in their facilities. Moreover, about 15% of NAViGO employees have experience of mental health problems and many still use services periodically. In the author's previous career, services well-meaningly, if somewhat paternalistically, kept secrets they thought might be upsetting from people who used services and sometimes from staff too. We try hard not to do this, have complete openness within the bounds of clinical confidentiality and to many of us older staff, the more this is done, the better and more comfortable it becomes. I often wonder why I didn't always do this, when the only downside is ensuring all things are explained in ways that can be understood by all. That can be time-consuming sometimes, but again a good discipline. This culture has led to many schemes, designs and initiatives coming directly from people who use services and many excellent debates too. It also makes people like myself confident of performing my role for the organisation. For readers' benefit, we are not discussing a service for a select group here. The services run include statutory mental health and associated social care services, including all acute mental health services.

Valued Roles

These can be anything that help people to be seen in positive ways. Within NAViGO some of the main changes were moving away from more traditional day services, to activities that allowed people to gain new skills, explore, gain qualifications, work experiences and indeed work within the organisation, moving towards future employment outside of the organisation also. 'Tukes', named after William Tuke (29), a man radically ahead of his time and a mental health pioneer, is the generic name for all NAViGO's employment, training and work experience schemes. They started by turning over all our own ancillary services to this cause, by doing all our own catering, cleaning, maintenance, horticulture, laundry and so forth in this way. This indeed produced a double virtue; people becoming re-motivated, working inside and outside the NAViGO services and gaining skills, qualifications and structure in their lives and, in tandem, the service gained flexible top quality provision, often better respected by those using services and staffing them because of their involvement. Ninety percent plus scores for cleaning are the norm now (they had hit an all-time low of 35% with a private cleaning company previously), and the sense of togetherness and community is second to none. NAViGO facilities are often commented on as hotel quality, and if I need a shelf put up today I can have that done. Not only that, but also the shelf I actually want will be put up, not one from NHS supplies in the wrong colour! Extending this scheme further, NAViGO runs shops, cafes, a full-sized commercial garden centre bought on the open market, a local park and many other schemes that both connect people to the public and help them be seen in valued roles. Here is a virtuous circle; such schemes also generate some income, and in this way, the extras the members want over and above statutory requirements funded by taxation can be financed directly by the public through trading. Indeed, the public very often vocally support this service.

Human Factors in Unit Design

Most staff, if asked, would intuitively say that acute units are often too big. In the author's career they have gone from 40 or more beds as the norm, to mid to low 20s. An improved milieu, reduced conflict, and more independence and individuality can be expected from even smaller units. If you still wish to keep people doing daily routines like supported cooking and maintaining their dietary needs, then numbers need to be smaller and facilities more domestic in size and appearance. The standard acute unit model often removes people's ability to do anything much for themselves and creates rapid dependence.

Even when very unwell, people should arguably not be allowed to simply switch off. They can, with help, invariably maintain some involvement for themselves. These times, too, provide excellent ability for interaction, connection, therapeutic intervention and assessment. So why not have units with ten beds? The answer generally, where it has been thought through and considered, is issues of logistics and cost. Redesign of teams and work makes it possible for NAViGO to work with ten-bed units. They have open-plan kitchens and very discrete security features to avoid labelling. In-reach/outreach is with the same team covering the whole acute phase (unit, crisis and home treatment) as one caseload and staff moving where the need is greatest at any given time. There is also a flexible five-bed enhanced care unit, which is open or closed depending on need. This can be used for an hour or a few days. This design has meant vastly decreased use of beds and much shorter stays. People who use the service rate it much higher than average nationally (85%+ good or excellent). Even more impressive has been the reduction in average length of stay from 58 days to 22 days and occupancy rates from 138% to 92% with fewer overall beds. At the same time people's rating of the quality of care has risen dramatically. Another feature is a vastly reduced use of Psychiatric Intensive Care Unit beds.

Older People's 'Home from Home'

More recently, in response to the very poor outcomes and sad reports of neglect of older people within general hospital environments, another scheme has emerged. The scheme called 'home from home' looks to address some of the problems recently highlighted. It aims to provide successful and dignified care for older people with confusion due to or associated with physical illness. This service is run in partnership with the general hospital and seeks to create the right environment, staff team and flexibility to fully address people's treatment and care needs. The previous problem was that an older person admitted to a general ward with complex needs and confusion would get appropriate medical treatment but in an environment which prejudiced overall outcomes. The general hospital ward is simply not designed for confused people, who may need to wander and because they cannot do so safely in that environment may end up being sedated. What follows is loss of independence and this may lead to institutional placement afterwards. Home from home is a bespoke in-reach/outreach service with the same team managing 15 community and 15 bed places. The service has all the mental health and physical health skills and a connection with social care. It is able to consider and meet needs appropriately. Carers can be admitted with the person receiving care, which increases familiarity and possibilities for self-care. The bespoke environment allows wandering but encourages rest and also social functioning. Facilities allow self-support as much as possible and admissions are shorter and less traumatic. Best of all, the vast majority of people using the service go back to their normal place of residence, mostly due to a healthier balance between treatment need and other care and human factors. We break no spirits!

The Future of SRV-Based Modelling

So what of the future of this style of thinking in stimulating models and gaining a better balance in overall services? The author believes many old models need refreshing to gain a better equilibrium.

Let us consider the perennial issues of people with serious mental illness (SMI) suffering preventable physical illness (mostly due to poor diet and lifestyle problems) and older people being isolated, as examples. A standard health response, which is partially successful, is to physically monitor people with SMI and refer to GPs whilst trying to encourage sports clubs and other activities. There is nothing wrong with these activities, but they are limited in effect. Just imagine being told you have an SMI in your youth and probably being signed off sick. Eighty-seven percent of people with SMI are unemployed and they are by far the most discriminated against group in the work arena. You might then be asked to attend a day hospital, and be given medications that stimulate your appetite and, sadly as a side effect, sometimes dull your motivation. You will not be allowed to drive and often, sadly, friendships and relationships may fracture too. With no real role and little hope, you may become more demotivated, without transport spending more time at home and possibly eating more take-away and convenience foods. It is a pattern many follow almost inevitably.

Now consider older people and isolation, depression and lack of supervision and activity. The biggest cause of admission to hospital with confusion, when audited before Home from Home, was dehydration. Again a standard response might be to refer the person to a voluntary agency for a lunch club or similar. Sadly, many of these social interventions have been subject to considerable reduction in the current austerity in public services. Even if available, is a free lunch what is needed? The elderly person may be grateful for something to relieve the isolation but may feel demeaned. Why would you give me charity? Am I worthy of that now? Can I do anything in return to preserve my pride and make me feel useful/needed?

The answer then may be completely non-traditional, if using SRV as the lens through which to look at these issues. Why not a community supermarket? Yes, a real supermarket selling all the things supermarkets do, but with a different emphasis. Where we all shop together, no food banks for the poor, or subsidised shops where only the poor or disadvantaged groups can be (ever stood in the free school dinners queue?). A supermarket where the profits from you and I are put back and subsidise people like those with SMI who have dietary problems, to help them gain healthy habits and use foods better. Where you can prescribe, as part of early interventions, a subsidised healthy diet and cooking skills. Better still, where older people at risk of isolation can come and share their best recipes with such young people and be engaged with helping them gain better understandings of diet. Those isolated people have then rightly earned a lunch and whilst we are here let's have a rollicking good sing-along too, you've earned it! Where the profits from the community's shopping are reinvested in the community and many other community functions take place, too, in a more social setting. And yes of course work, training, skills and education for vulnerable groups would be present too, but nobody would know who was who, who was subsidised and who was just passing through shopping. That, in a time of austerity particularly, when the message is clear that government doesn't wish to pay more for health, is the way to make services valuable to the public and remove the stigma of receiving them. It is the author's view that most people wouldn't mind paying more for health services. They just don't want to finance the huge and seemingly out-of-touch bureaucracy that creates all the stigma and separation in the first place.

So, thinking in terms of valued roles and really tackling problems, I do not wish my role to be a recipient of charity, or simply that of patient. I need to be more! Let's insist on the services that we offer to disadvantaged groups being what we might expect for a family member. Let's insist on the services being organised to offer people a sense of value, at very least not damaging what they already have.

Further, let's design things to consider how people as recipients will likely be seen by others. Victims? Of less importance? Harmless in need of charity? Potentially dangerous and in need of greater security? Unable to take any decisions for themselves?

Primum non nocere and let us have a revolution where the dimensions of spirit, pride, soul and the way people will be perceived by others are given a prominent place in all our designs of service, way beyond the dictates of simple functionality, or just a passing nod to aesthetic issues.

References

1. NHS Providers/Healthcare Financial Management Association. Funding mental health at local level – unpicking the variation. 2016. Available at: nhsproviders.org/resource-library/reports/funding-mental-health-at-local-level-unpicking-the-variation (accessed 12/9/16).
2. Whitbourne SK. The essential guide to defense mechanisms – can you spot your favourite form of deception? *Psychology Today*. 2011. Available at: psychologytoday.com/blog/fulfillment-any-age/201110/the-essential-guide-defense-mechanisms. (accessed 12/9/16).
3. Cory P. Stigma shout. 2008. Mental Health Media/Mind/Rethink. Available at: time-to-change.org.uk/sites/default/files/Stigma%20Shout.pdf (accessed 12/9/16).
4. Henderson C, Noblett J, Parke H, Clement S, Caffrey A, Gale-Grant O, Shultze B, Druss B, Thornicroft G. Mental health-related stigma in health care and mental health-care settings. *Lancet*. 2014; 1(6):467–482.
5. Thornicroft G. Physical health disparities and mental illness: the scandal of premature mortality. *British Journal of Psychiatry*. 2011; 199(6):441–442.
6. Wattis J, Curran S. Spirituality and mental well being in old age. *Geriatric Medicine*. 2006; 36(12):13–17.
7. Rogers M, Wattis J. Spirituality in nursing practice *Nursing Standard*. 2015; 29(39):51–57.
8. Jones J, Topping A, Wattis J, Smith J. A concept analysis of spirituality in occupational therapy practice. *Journal for the Study of Spirituality*. 2016; 6(1):1–20.
9. Gilburt H. Trust finances raise concerns about the future of the Mental Health Taskforce recommendations. The Kings Fund. 2016. Available at: https://www.kingsfund.org.uk/blog/2016/10/trust-finances-mental-health-taskforce (accessed 3/2/2017).
10. Royal College of Psychiatrists. Whole-person care: From rhetoric to reality – achieving parity between mental and physical health. *Occasional paper OP* 88. 2013. Available at: rcpsych.ac.uk/pdf/OP88.pdf (accessed 15/9/16).
11. Allan C. The most toxic issue facing those with mental health problems is stigma. *Guardian Society*. 2013. Available at: theguardian.com/society/2013/apr/03/mental-health-problems-stigma-employers (accessed 15/9/16).
12. Corrigan P. How stigma interferes with mental health care. *American Psychologist*. 2004; 59(7):614–625.
13. Wolfensberger W. Social role valorization: a proposed new term for the principle of normalization. *Mental Retardation*. 1983; 21(6):234–239.
14. Flynn RJ, Lemay RA (eds.). A Quarter Century of Normalization and Social Role Valorization: Evolution and Impact. Ottawa: University of Ottawa Press; 1999.
15. Thomas S, Wolfensberger W. An overview of social role valorization. In Flynn, RJ, Lemay RA (eds.). *A Quarter Century of Normalization and Social Role Valorization: Evolution and Impact*. Ottawa: University of Ottawa Press; 1999.
16. Purkiss J. Socially valued roles: a reflection. 2015. Weblog. Available at: jeanettepurkis.com (accessed 15/9/16).
17. Osburn J. An overview of Social Role Valorization theory. *The SRV Journal*. 2006; 1(1):4–13.

18. Goffman E. Asylums: Essays on the Social Situation of Mental Patients and Other Inmates. Garden City, NY: Anchor Books; 1961.

19. Lammers S, Verhey A. *On Moral Medicine: Theological Perspectives in Medical Ethics* (2nd edition). Chicago: Wm. B. Eerdmans Publishing; 1998.

20. Francis R. Report of the Mid Staffordshire NHS Foundation Trust Public Inquiry. London: The Stationery Office; 2013.

21. McGarty C, Yzerbyt VY, Spears R. Social, Cultural and Cognitive Factors in Stereotype Formation. Stereotypes as Explanations: The Formation of Meaningful Beliefs About Social Groups. Cambridge: Cambridge University Press; 2002.

22. Anderson ML, Taylor HF. *Sociology: The Essentials*. Belmont, CA: Wadsworth; 2009.

23. World Health Organization. The world health report 2001 - Mental Health: New Understanding, New Hope. Press release: Mental disorders affect one in four people. 2001. Available at: who.int/whr/2001/media_centre/press_release/en (accessed 15/9/16).

24. Inman T. Foundation for a new theory and practice of medicine. John Churchill, 1860. Cited in: Sokol DK, First do no harm revisited. *British Medical Journal*. 2013; 347:f6426.

25. Papoulias C, Csipke E, Rose D, McKellar S, Wykes T. The psychiatric ward as a therapeutic space: systematic review. *The British Journal of Psychiatry*. 2014; 205 (3):171–176.

26. Meehan T. The careful nursing philosophy and professional practice model. *Journal of Clinical Nursing*. 2012; 21(19):2905–2916.

27. Jacobson N, Greenley D. What is recovery? A conceptual model and explication. *Psychiatric Services*. 2001; 52(4):482–485.

28. Slay J, Stephens L. *Co-Production in Mental Health: A Literature Review*. London: New Economics Foundation; 2013.

29. Bewley T. Madness to Mental Illness. A History of the Royal College of Psychiatrists. London: Royal College of Psychiatrists; 2008.

A Vision for the Future **13**

John Wattis, Stephen Curran and Melanie Rogers

A Joy and an Inspiration

Assembling the chapters for this book has been a joy and an inspiration. The inspiration has come from seeing authors from many different backgrounds wrestling so successfully with the issues of spiritually competent practice. The joy has come from realising how much we have in common and how the themes expressed by our authors come together and interact to make a coherent whole. Authors come from a variety of disciplines and religious/non-religious backgrounds but all are concerned with putting spiritual needs and issues at the forefront of practice in health and social care. We hope we have made the case that describing spiritually competent practice (rather than wrangling over a precise definition for spirituality) is the starting point for improving practice. Our authors have identified cultural and organisational obstacles to spiritually competent care but have also reported examples of how those obstacles can be overcome at a cultural, organisational and personal level.

Our organisational cultures need to change and educational institutions can help by educating clinicians and managers to enable them to recognise and implement the changes needed. The secular materialism of the *modern age* combined with the associated reductionist approach to science tends to discount mind (except as an epiphenomenon) and has even less time for concepts like spirit (see Chapter 6). In the *post-modern age* people are grappling with the ancient question 'What is truth?' We would boldly assert the truth that human beings are spiritual beings in the sense that they seek meaning, purpose and value in life and are more than just biological mechanisms to be overhauled like a car engine when 'faulty'. This truth is recognised in terms like whole-person, holistic or spiritually competent care. What spiritually competent care adds to the other terms is to emphasise the aspect of holistic care that is perhaps most often neglected – the fact that human beings are creatures who seek to find meaning, purpose and connectedness with other people (and perhaps with the transcendental or sacred). The human search for meaning is expressed in the narratives we construct for ourselves individually and as a society.

We need an approach to health and social care that values the humanity of the people who receive care and of the people who provide it, recognising that they ideally work together in partnership. We have a capacity for empathy and relationship and a need to make sense of our lives and be valued that marks us out as living human beings. There is an overlap between person-centred care, spiritually competent care, compassionate care, intelligent kindness and mindful compassion. We do not need to fight about terminology. Truly person-centred care will inevitably involve the spirit. Spiritual care, compassionate care, intelligent kindness and mindful compassion can all be regarded as inspired by our common humanity. We need to respect this common humanity and not simply see the people we serve as a means to an end of reaching arbitrary 'targets'. And we need to change organisational systems that tend to drive the humanity out of health and care staff (Chapters 10, 11 and 12 give examples of how this can be done). We live in a culture where 'the powers that be' seem more interested in numbers and appearances than real human experience, especially in the experience of those who are not wealthy in the material sense. We need to resist the dehumanising pressures this culture fosters.

All of us who value humanity and the search for meaning, irrespective of whether we frame this in religious language or not, may find ourselves at odds with a dominant culture that sees people mainly as potential sources of financial gain rather than human beings who seek a purpose for their lives in meaningful work, relationships and sometimes enduring suffering (1). Here we examine some of the common themes that have emerged in this book, looking especially at the dominant worldview in the West and the importance of treating patients as people, not as technical 'problems' to be solved. We look also at some of the obstacles to developing a spiritually competent health service and outline how we can enable real change through cultural shift at a personal and organisational level. We also outline the educational and research effort needed to underpin this change.

The Dominant Worldview in the West

The Western worldview and culture is secular, materialistic, individualistic and often accepts gross inequality between people as inevitable or even desirable. Its (secular) 'religion' could be described as economism (2). This worldview has been consistently challenged by writers on management and leadership. Some examples follow.

Charles Handy, philosopher and management expert writing over 20 years ago, explored the dissatisfaction that the pursuit of technology and market economics could bring. In his book *The Empty Raincoat* (3), he wrote:

> What is happening in our mature societies is much more fundamental, confusing and distressing than I had expected… Part of the confusion stems from out pursuit of efficiency and economic growth, in the conviction that these are the necessary ingredients of progress. In pursuit of these goals we can be tempted to forget that it is we, individual men and women, who should be the measure of all things, not made to measure for something else. It is easy to lose ourselves in efficiency, to treat that efficiency as an end in itself and not a means to other ends (3, p.1).

Handy admits he does not have all the answers but he asks highly relevant questions about the emptiness that many people experience in our materialistic society. Citing Vaclav Havel, the first president of the Czech Republic, he argues moreover for a respect for something beyond ourselves and for a 'superpersonal' moral order without which we will not be able to create the social structures in which a person can truly be a person.

A decade later Steven Covey (4) found much the same dissatisfaction and argued that what was needed was a 'paradigm shift', a shift in the basic assumptions underlying Western culture. He suggested that this could be achieved if individuals used the freedom they possessed to choose a better way, accept what he described as 'universal principles' and express their voice, changing themselves (and their work colleagues and organisations) in the process.

In 2012, after the banking crisis, Gary Hamel (5) also argued that we needed to rethink the fundamental assumptions we have about management, the meaning of work and organisational life. He argued for a new vision for business leadership based on better principles and moral values, innovation, adaptability and passionate commitment.

There are good academic arguments that the rising inequality that results from our current culture is not good for personal or social health. These were eloquently expressed in the book *The Spirit Level* (6) where the authors demonstrated that, once a certain minimum level of national wealth had been achieved, physical and mental health and a variety of social problems, ranging from rates of imprisonment to teenage pregnancy, were all worse in more unequal societies. The film based on this book, *The Great Divide* (7), dramatized the consequences of inequality, especially in British and American Society.

Perhaps the first step in providing spiritually competent care is to recognise that the society we live in does need to change. As a society we must acknowledge that all people need to be treated with compassion and respect and that mechanistic, industrialised models of care and management are not appropriate in health and social care. The authors of Chapter 2 point out that any culture is in a state of flux and this applies with particular force to many elements of modern Western culture. Those who really want to see a better, more humane approach to health and social care need to become agents for change and to steer themselves and their organisations in that direction. As Mahatma Gandhi said:

Be the change you want to see in the world.

How do we do this? First we need to agree our underlying assumptions; our principles and values. The authors of the chapters in this book have written a great deal about the importance of relating to people who use our services as people, not objects to be processed. In the next section we explore this a bit further. Then we look at the organisational and cultural obstacles to achieving this. Finally, we explore how we can make these aspirations real. It can be done.

Organisational Obstacles to Spiritually Competent Care in Western Culture

One recurrent theme from many of our authors is the need for staff to have the time, the space and the skills to address spiritual needs. A culture in which professional values and ethics are discounted and care fragmented in favour of industrialised models of provision also makes spiritually competent care more difficult.

Strictly rationed interventions may mean that a professional has to stop working with the person she is supporting before she judges it to be appropriate from a professional point of view and perhaps just before a 'breakthrough' is achieved in the person's recovery. Incentive schemes, targets and performance indicators tend to reward that which is easy to measure, but as sociologist William Bruce Cameron wrote in the 1960s, '... not everything that can be counted counts, and not everything that counts can be counted' (8, p.13).

Sometimes attempts not to 'breach' numerical targets (e.g. waiting time in accident and emergency [A&E] departments) can lead to 'solutions' that amount to 'playing the game' rather than improving the quality of patient care. That is not to say such targets are always useless, but great caution needs to be exercised if they are used as a basis for financial incentives (or disincentives). The important thing about performance indicators is how they are interpreted. The waiting time in A&E may be a result of under-staffing, a major emergency diverting staff or the unavailability of inpatient care beds or social services support. Likewise, shortage of trained staff on wards may be due to lack of funding, failure to train sufficient numbers of clinicians due to political decisions made years ago, and so forth. In these circumstances blaming and shaming the clinical staff or their managers only destroys morale and does nothing to improve performance.

You may wonder what this has to do with spirituality. In fact, an obsession with what can be counted, micro-management, politically-driven targets and a failure to look for the reason(s) behind any apparent 'underperformance' set up a culture which is inimical to spiritually competent care. Staff deemed to be underperforming when the fault really lies elsewhere, are also likely to become demoralised and, as noted in Chapter 7, lack of opportunity to provide compassionate, person-centred care may be one of the factors leading to professional burn-out, which is equated in Chapter 6 with 'spiritual depletion'. Behind all this obsession with what can be counted is the reductionist, secular materialist worldview discussed above which can lead industrial 'mechanical' models of care and management that leave no room for person-centred, spiritually competent care. No amount of tinkering at the edges can change this fundamental reality. The current fashion in England for 'integrated care' and the Sustainability and Transformation Plan (9) cannot in themselves deliver the fundamental paradigm change that Covey (4, p.19) argues is necessary. Below we give some ideas of what is needed to achieve such a radical shift. This we believe would be of great benefit not only to people who use health services but also to people who provide and manage them.

Making it Real

Being Fully Human

The 'industrial' model of care often results in a bad experience for the people who use our services. It treats them as objects to be 'fixed' rather than as fellow human beings who need help and with whom practitioners are privileged to share a challenging (if often small) part of life's journey. There is an ethical imperative to be person-centred. From this imperative flows a whole range of consequences. We need to focus on the whole person, often in the context of their family or other caregivers. We need actively to seek their point of view and listen to their stories in order to identify what is important to them. We need to recognise the personal strengths and resources they each bring to the situation. Practitioners have expertise in specialized areas but the people who use our services are the experts in their own lives. We must recognise this and work in partnership with them. The narrative approach, discussed in Chapter 4, emphasises the benefits of recognising people as experts in their own lives.

Recognising people's right to self-determination involves making sure we have heard their point of view and concerns by listening carefully. Equally it means that we have ensured that they understand, as fully as possible, any choices that we put before them. We must support people in finding resources (internal as well as external) to help them cope with and understand the challenges that face them, rather than focus solely on the service imperatives that we are driven by. This applies particularly to people with conditions like dementia where extra effort is needed to involve them personally as far as possible. On occasion we may even have to recognise our own right to self-determination and refuse to be driven by inappropriate organisational imperatives.

Researching and practicing in this field, one becomes aware of 'work-arounds' that clinicians develop to mitigate the dehumanising effects of some organisational policies. Of course, professional boundaries have to be respected but there may be room for some flexing and appropriate sharing of personal experience as discussed in Chapter 4 and elsewhere. One of the authors of this chapter (JW) remembers how relieved an older female patient was when he reassured her that he did not think her charismatic Christian experiences were pathological because he had personally known many very sane charismatic Christians.

Perhaps the most important issue of all, in the area of treating people as people, is the issue of supporting people who are undervalued by society as a whole to realise their true value. People with severe mental illness, people with any long-standing illness or disability and older people are often devalued in a society which puts a premium on youth and material wealth or earning capacity. Chapters 11 and 12 tackle the issue of marginalised and devalued groups head on.

Concepts of person-centred care recur throughout this book. Empathy, warmth, genuineness and similar words are used frequently and link to concepts like hospitality, availability and vulnerability discussed especially in Chapter 4 and reprised in Chapter 9. They also link to other ideas like compassionate care (supported in NHS England by documents like Compassion in Practice (10), *Intelligent Kindness* (11) and *Mindful Compassion* (12). People can be educated in these principles but to truly embrace them requires self-awareness, making time for reflective practice and continuing personal transformation. Practitioners need to be fully present and able to form connections with the people they serve. This is not easy, and we also need to transform education, continuing professional development and staff support if this kind of change is to become pervasive and embedded in everyday practice.

Making this paradigm change real demands, as Covey suggests, that each of us 'finds our voice' (4, p.27). He sees two divergent possibilities for each of us. One is what he describes as the 'broad, well-travelled road to mediocrity', the other as 'the road to meaning and greatness'. The easy road is imposed from the outside in. It is simply to take on the 'cultural software' of our society, losing our voice (at the same time perhaps keeping others from finding their voice) and resulting in under-achievement. The other he describes as 'inside out' (remember the integrated model of spirituality discussed in Chapter 1). This uses our innate human creativity to help us find our voice (and others to find theirs) resulting in a truly meaningful life. In this context it is helpful to note that the two chapters on organisations that have achieved a measure of spiritual competence (Chapters 11 and 12) both emphasise creativity, one explicitly and the other implicitly through social role valorisation. There are also echoes of the idea of vocation advanced in Chapter 10. Choosing the road to meaning and using our creative abilities to move forward reminds us of Robert Frost's great poem *The Road Not Taken,* which ends:

> Two roads diverged in a wood, and I—
> I took the one less traveled by,
> And that has made all the difference (13).

The Road Less Traveled was used as the title for M. Scott Peck's best-selling work first published in 1978 and re-issued in 2006 (14), giving a psychotherapist's viewpoint on what he described as 'a new psychology of love, traditional values, and spiritual growth'.

Organisational and Cultural Facilitators

If the starting point for spiritually competent practice is spiritual self-awareness, organisational awareness of spirituality comes a close second. Without this the spiritually competent practitioner finds herself constantly having to work around (or even against) the system, rather than with it. We have discussed two organisations with a measure of spiritual awareness in earlier chapters. Both are marked by what we would call 'devolved creativity'. In the NAViGO project this is explicitly based on the concept of social role valorisation. The principles employed can be briefly summarised as

- Have people who use and work in services influence how they are designed and operated.
- Design facilities on a domestic scale (and, in mental health, domestic in style, too).
- Education of staff to help them understand their power and influence for good or bad.
- Ensure that organisational design focuses on the needs of people who use it.
- Language is important. Use the word 'people' a lot. Avoid clinical language and shorthand that creates distance rather than connection.
- Involve people who know – the people who use the services – in all training of staff.
- Make clinical and security features unobtrusive to avoid unnecessary 'distance'.
- Share as much common space as possible between people who use and work in the service.
- Encourage public access to break down the social stigma of mental health issues, create opportunities for positive interaction with the local community.
- Support people (staff and service users) to develop valued roles, springing loose their creativity.

This could be summed up as co-creating conditions that maximise the opportunity for person-to-person connection, thus supporting the value of the individual. The end result in NAViGO has been very productive with a wealth of innovative projects led by people who use and work in the services *and feel valued.* Despite the severe financial constraints imposed by an economic climate of austerity, the organisation has achieved a great deal.

The other organisation (SWYFT, Chapter 11) is much bigger than NAViGO and has channelled creativity through the Creative Minds and Spirit in Mind projects. These use specialised staff to co-create amazing projects that have supported people, alongside more conventional services, and begun to build links with local faith communities. Even though the underlying philosophy appears different, relating to developing the creative ability of people who use (and provide) services, the end results are not dissimilar. People feel valued and able to contribute, connections and friendships are developed and people find meaning and purpose in life.

Team-working and good leadership are vital organisational facilitators. As illustrated in Chapter 10, effort put into team-building in hospice, and recognising that everyone has a role in spiritual care reaps rewards. Other organisations need to invest in team-building and the organisational stability needed to make it possible. This is in opposition to the political tendency to promote repeated reorganisation. Ideally, multi-disciplinary teams should have a stable membership and be educated together about person-centred, compassionate, spiritually competent care. Charles Handy, in *The Gods of Management* (15), uses analogies with the Greek gods to describe four different management cultures: Zeus presides over the *club culture*, Apollo over the *role culture*, Athena over the *task culture* and Dionysius over the *existential (or craft) culture*. Zeus makes fast decisions, often from the top of relatively small enterprises, and works by networking at a senior level. Apollo is the god of order who defines staff through their job descriptions and not as individuals – as long as you get attention from the right grade of staff, it doesn't matter who they are. Staff are interchangeable cogs in the machine and control is top-down. This fits the industrial and mechanical styles of management described and criticised earlier. It is good for pre-defined, steady-state tasks like running payroll, but out of place in solving problems or coping with change. Handy, originally writing toward the end of the 20th century, described an 'Apollonian crisis' in many organisations. The present-day health service still suffers from too much Apollonian management, sadly reinforced by inspection regimes. Athena, the warrior goddess, recognises expertise and solves problems. Clinical teams often work for Athena, problem-solving with people and coping with the unexpected. Dionysus creates a culture where staff essentially work semi-independently and owe little allegiance to management. Each style of management has its place but the problem-solving, expertise-sharing team tends to be most effective at the clinical level (and possibly in managing large organisations too). Building and maintaining clinical teams, helping them to become person-centred and facilitating spiritually competent care is a key leadership task. Good leaders need to be equally concerned with the task at hand and the people who deliver and use the services. They need to create conditions in which staff can, in turn, use their own specialised knowledge, skills and creativity to achieve success. The alternative is to attempt to micromanage in a bureaucratic way, and this seems doomed to failure. Clinical staff also need to co-create solutions with the people who use their services. For a more detailed discussion of these issues, see *Practical Management and Leadership for Doctors* (16).

Organisations can also facilitate spiritually competent practice (and good practice generally) by having realistic expectations of what staff can achieve and by providing time, space and support to front-line practitioners. Managers need to understand the relational aspect of good practice and understand that breaking up care into discrete tasks, each performed by different people, may make healing relationships more difficult to sustain. Creating 'an environment in which clinical excellence can flourish' (17) means creating the conditions in which staff have the time, motivation and competency to deliver good interpersonal care as well as handling the technical aspects of care.

Educational and Developmental Facilitators of Spiritually Competent Practice

One of the most consistent findings in this area is that nurses and other practitioners often feel ill-prepared to address spiritual needs (see Chapter 5). Preparing students to practice competently in the area of spirituality involves much more than teaching knowledge and skills. One of the prerequisites of good practice in this area is spiritual self-awareness. Developing this requires special approaches to teaching, as discussed in Chapters 1 and 5 and elsewhere. Self-awareness, reflective learning, sharing and modelling by clinical teachers, and the basics of the person-centred approach are central to this approach. In addition, an understanding of how illness can challenge the personal narratives that people develop to give meaning and purpose to their lives is needed, coupled with a willingness to provide support as people address these challenges. Educators working in this area report finding themselves working more on a level with their students (18). In technical areas their expertise may be much greater than that of their students but in being human we can all potentially learn from each other.

Just as service providers need to create time and space for practitioners to attend to the spiritual needs of the people they serve, so also those who set standards and provide education for practitioners need to create time and space for learners in this area. Individual educators can only do a so much if the importance of the more interpersonal aspects of practice is not recognised by educational institutions.

At the postgraduate level, spiritually competent practice can be encouraged and supported by discussion in the multidisciplinary team setting, through continuing professional development (often also conducted on an interdisciplinary basis) and by supervision, coaching and mentoring. Peer supervision and mentoring, and peer groups to support continuing professional development can add to this.

Research and Development

In business and industry, research and development (R&D) commonly go hand in hand. If someone designs a more efficient way of delivering the fuel–air mixture into the combustion chamber of a car engine it is likely over time that engines will be redesigned to accommodate this. This, in fact, happened when the carburetor largely gave way to fuel injection. In clinical practice, research on new treatments is implemented (often imperfectly) through clinical guidelines and cost–benefit analyses conducted through agencies such as the National Institute for Health and Clinical Excellence (NICE; 19). However, when it comes to management practice (and sometimes political policy) there is a tendency to follow fashion rather than evidence. Even where is evidence, there is a notorious knowing-doing gap. Pfeffer and Sutton made a detailed study of this and came to a number of interesting conclusions (20). Their first principle is that knowing by doing ensures there is no gap between what is known and what is done. This is stated succinctly in the aphorism 'practice makes perfect'. This also reflects another of their conclusions that reading books (even this one), having presentations and holding meetings about change (even when those meetings make a positive decision to change) does not, *of itself*, produce change. They make many other interesting observations including the role of organisational memory and culture in preventing implementation of new ideas. Even organisations that focus on knowledge management tend to view knowledge as intellectual property to be placed in a repository rather than a resource to be used. This also happens to academic research.

So, the first thing to say about research and development is that we need to put what we already know from existing research into practice. There is a considerable body of research into different areas of spirituality in health and health care, some of it reviewed in chapters in this book, but more needs to be done, and some of the most substantial quantitative findings have measured religious practice, which is only an imperfect surrogate for spirituality. These have been briefly reviewed by Koenig in his helpful guide *Spirituality in Patient Care* (21, pp.22–30).

As discussed in Chapter 1, spirituality is a concept which has broadened and changed in its meaning over time. Originally it was used to describe the person with deep inner religious experience and was almost synonymous with the term 'mystical' (see Chapter 1). More recently it has expanded to describe the human quest for meaning and purpose. Spiritual well-being likewise is seen by some as an existential phenomenon related to the psychological concepts of well-being. Koenig (22) questioned the use of the term *spirituality* in research because instruments used to measure spirituality reflected this wider meaning. He found these measures to be heavily 'contaminated' with questions assessing positive character traits or mental health. This had the not unexpected effect that spirituality measured by these instruments correlated with good mental health. Koenig argued that this was tautological and that, for research purposes, spirituality should be defined and measured in traditional terms or abandoned. He also argued elsewhere (21, p.38) that spirituality was a useful broad term for clinicians when talking with patients, some of who may not consider themselves religious.

Part of the issue here is the use of appropriate research methods. Qualitative research may be better able to address the kind of questions that spirituality raises. Janice Jones, co-author of two chapters in this book, researched how spiritual care was delivered in occupational therapy practice. Her findings were based on observational studies of practice and interviews with the occupational therapists observed. It is worth quoting at some length from the abstract of her doctoral thesis:

> Despite the difficulties defining spirituality occupational therapists appeared able to apply the underpinning core values and philosophy of the profession and embed spirituality in their practice. Practitioners found it more meaningful to describe spirituality in terms of how they applied the concept in, and through, practice by comprehending the values, needs and concerns of the individual as opposed to a consistent definition. Occupational therapists engaged with spirituality by concerning themselves with supporting patients experiencing vulnerability due to disruption in their health and well-being. This support was achieved by the occupational therapist uncovering the individual needs of the patient and through delivering person-centred care by explicitly addressing spirituality. The scope to embed spirituality was on occasion limited by organisational and contextual factors that restricted the potential to practice fully. Achieving organisational targets by adopting time constrained interventions was perceived as having a particularly limiting impact on embedding spirituality in practice (23).

These findings, like Carl Rogers' original findings on client-centred therapy and the whole person-centred movement discussed in Chapter 1, depend on observational, qualitative research. Qualitative research is particularly suited to exploring meaning and therefore a vital tool in research into spiritually competent practice.

Melanie Rogers and Laura Béres, in Chapter 4, have also shown how concepts such as hospitality, availability and vulnerability and the understanding and use of narrative can be used in developing understanding of and implementing spiritually competent care. Quantitative scientists will immediately ask themselves whether scales can be developed to measure such variables in the same way that Carl Rogers' principles of empathy, non-possessive warmth and genuineness have been measured. Perhaps they can. In any case there is enormous scope for further research in the area of how spiritually competent care can be taught and put into practice.

There is also need for research in the area of how organisations can foster spiritually competent practice. Current knowledge suggests that first moves should be from an industrial to a more personal focus for care and that adequate support of staff helps enable them to provide truly holistic care. Then there is the question of the spirituality of organisations, which can be viewed as a metaphor for what gives the organisation meaning, purpose, motivation and values. This is partly addressed in Giacalone and Jurkeiewicz's *Handbook of Workplace Spirituality and Organizational Performance* (24) but this is still an area begging for more research, especially in health care, because the evidence seems to suggest that the spirit of the organisation is very important in obstructing or facilitating spiritually competent care.

Conclusion

In this book we have sought to inspire our readers about the relevance of spirituality in health care. We recognise that spirituality is more diverse in definition and more difficult to express in quantitative terms than religion or religious practice. We have wrestled with the issue of how we define spirituality and concluded that describing spiritually competent practice does not depend on a precise definition of spirituality and is therefore more useful in practice. Our authors have examined how our dominant Western culture predisposes us to dismiss the importance of spirituality or to make the issue so intensely personal that it is impossible to draw general conclusions. Different approaches to addressing spiritual needs and developing spiritually competent practice have been discussed. Organisational issues have been considered and we have presented examples of good practice that can transform individuals and organisations. Authors have considered issues relating to spiritually competent practice in acute care, primary care, mental health and end of life care. We have stressed the importance of organisational support for staff to facilitate spiritually competent practice and suggested what educational approaches might best help develop and sustain competent practice.

If you agree that this is an important area for practice, for education and for research, it is over to you. Our authors are all involved in one way or another in spiritually competent practice, research and/or education in this area. We encourage all our readers to increase the attention they pay to spirituality in practice and become the change we all want to see in improving how we support the people we are called to help.

References

1. Frankl V. *Man's Search for Meaning*. London: Rider Books; 2004.
2. Norgaard. The Church of Economism and Its Discontents. Great Transition Initiative website. 2015. Available at: greattransition.org/publication/the-church-of-economism-and-its-discontents (accessed 22/9/16).
3. Handy C. *The Empty Raincoat*. London: Arrow Books; 2002.
4. Covey S. *The 8th Habit*. London: Simon and Schuster; 2004.
5. Hamel G. *What Matters Now*. San Francisco: Jossey Bass; 2012.
6. Wilkinson R, Pickett K. *The Spirit Level*. London: Penguin Books; 2011.
7. Havey Productions. The Great Divide. 2015. Available at: vimeo.com/ondemand/thegreatdivide (accessed 22/9/16).
8. Cameron WB. *Informal Sociology, A Casual Introduction to Sociological Thinking*. New York: Random House; 1967.
9. NHS England. Sustainability and transformation plans. 2016. Available at: england.nhs.uk/ourwork/futurenhs/deliver-forward-view/stp (accessed 22/9/16).
10. NHS England. Compassion in Practice. 2012. Available at: england.nhs.uk/wp-content/uploads/2012/12/compassion-in-practice.pdf (accessed 22/9/16).
11. Ballat J, Campling P. *Intelligent Kindness: Reforming the Culture of Healthcare*. London: Royal College of Psychiatrists; 2011.
12. Gilbert P, Choden. *Mindful Compassion*. London: Robinson; 2013.
13. Frost R, Orr D (eds.). *The Road Not Taken and Other Poems* (Centenary edition). New York: Penguin; 2015.
14. Scott-Peck M. *The Road Less Traveled*. London: Arrow; 2007.
15. Handy C. *The Gods of Management*. London: Souvenir Press; 2009.
16. Wattis J, Curran S. *Practical Management and Leadership for Doctors*. London: CRC Press; 2011.
17. Scally G, Donaldson L. Clinical governance and the drive for quality improvement in the new NHS in England. *BMJ*. 1998; 317:61–65.
18. Prentis S, Rogers M, Wattis J, Jones J, Stephenson J. Healthcare lecturers' perceptions of spirituality in education. *Nursing Standard*. 2014; 29 (3):44–52.
19. National Institute for Health and Clinical Excellence. Available at: nice.org.uk (accessed 22/9/16).
20. Pfeffer J, Sutton R. *The Knowing-Doing Gap*. New York: Harvard Business Press; 1999.
21. Koenig H. *Spirituality in Patient Care* (3rd edition). Philadelphia and London: Templeton Foundation Press; 2013.
22. Koenig H. Concerns about measuring 'spirituality' in research. *The Journal of Nervous and Mental Disease*. 2008; 196(5):349–355.
23. Jones J. A qualitative study exploring how occupational therapists embed spirituality into their practice. Doctoral thesis, University of Huddersfield. 2016. Available at: eprints.hud.ac.uk/27857 (accessed 22/9/16).
24. Giacalone RA, Jurkeiewicz CL. *Handbook of Workplace Spirituality and Organizational Performance*. New York: M.E. Sharpe; 2010.

Index

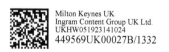